Persistent Remains Of The Foetal Hyaloid Artery

David DeBeck

AMERICAN OPHTHALMOLOGICAL MONOGRAPHS

No. 1.—October, 1890.

PERSISTENT REMAINS

OF THE

FOETAL HYALOID ARTERY

BY

DAVID DeBECK, M.D.

Assistant to the Chair of Ophthalmology, Medical College of Ohio; Member American Ophthalmological Society; Librarian Cincinnati Academy of Medicine

WITH TWELVE PLATES

CINCINNATI
PRESS OF ROBERT CLARKE & CO.
1890

A MONOGRAPH

OF THE

Congenital Anomalies and Hereditary Diseases

OF THE EYE.

VOL. III.

CHAPTER I.

ANOMALIES OF THE VITREOUS.

A—PERSISTENT HYALOID ARTERY.

The most important congenital anomaly of the vitreous humour is the persistence of some vestige of the hyaloid artery; a vessel which traverses this structure during fœtal life.

A cursory retrospect of this chapter in the development of the eye, will recall the salient points that are of essential import in this connection.

With the in-growth of the epiblast to form the crystalline lens, there coincides an involution of the primary optic vesicle to form the secondary optic vesicle, or optic cup, in the anterior opening of which the new lens rests. From the excentric direction of this involution, and from the more rapid growth forward and laterally of the top and sides of this optic cup, it remains open below :—the fœtal fissure. Through this fissure there passes in an off-shoot of the mesoblast to form the future vitreous. This process fills up this gap below, occupies a short space in the anterior part of the under groove of the optic stalk, which has begun to fold under laterally to form the future optic nerve, and fills out and soon enlarges the space between the lens and the hollow of the optic cup.

Coming forward from below and behind, an arterial twig from a mesoblastic branch passes into the eye. This is homologous (but variable), in all the Vertebrata. In the Mammalia it runs for a short distance in this groove on the inferior aspect of the optic stalk, and then passes forward into the vitreous. It gives some small provisional branches to supply the posterior portion of the vitreous, and then passes forward through the center of the vitreous toward the lens. It is surrounded by a fibrous sheath or adventitia of its own; by some authors it is said to lie free within an additional membranous tubular sheath, the canal of

Cloquet; by others the adventitia is regarded as its sole covering, and the canal traversed as simply a tubular, unlined passage-way through the vitreous. The latter view is hardly tenable.

Its course is usually straight, especially in the later stages of development when the vitreous is more completely developed; quite frequently it is sinuous, which seems the rule in the earlier stages when the vitreous is shallower; and rare instances have been noted where it twined into a distinct loop before reaching the lens. As a rule it remains a single trunk; although occasionally it may divide into two branches soon after leaving the optic stalk; and rarely it may subdivide into three or four branches, or even more when nearer the lens.

On reaching the posterior surface of the lens it divides and subdivides rapidly into a large number of smaller branches, which radiate in a stellate figure over the posterior surface of the lens, running toward its edge. These branches bend over the edge of the lens and many go to the vascular sheath forming a net-work on the anterior face of the lens, this sheath having been formed by in-growth of the mesoblast here. Thus a complete vascular envelope—the membrana capsulo-pupillaris—is formed to inclose and nourish the growing lens.

Many of these smaller branches of the hyaloid artery also anastomose with minute vessels, some of which are venous, around the anterior edge of the optic cup where the iris and ciliary body are being formed. These veins carry away the whole of the blood of this central vitreous artery, and not being necessary, it is never accompanied by a proper returning vein of its own.

The optic stalk completes its folding under and incloses the proximal portion of this vessel lying in its groove. It then is designated as the *arteria centralis retinae*; and from it grow out vessels to supply the retina. These, however, have nothing to do with the provisional earlier vessels of the vitreous. The fœtal fissure has long since closed below; the choroid and sclera are differentiated from layers of the mesoblast; the cornea is formed in front; and the eye begins to assume roughly its permanent form and structure.

The provisional vascular structures begin to be obliterated at the end of the fifth and the beginning of the sixth month of gestation. The hyaloid artery, hitherto red and carrying blood, becomes empty and white a short distance behind the lens. Its caliber becomes thinner and thinner, and finally its separates, either from the lens, or at some point in its anterior half. The filament attached to the lens gradually fades away, and the branches over the posterior face of the lens become finer and dimmer, and are rapidly absorbed. The posterior end shrivels up soon after. Examined now, a pyramidal process will be found, with its base covering the optic nerve, and its rapidly narrowing conical point projecting a short distance into the vitreous. This can be readily separated from the vitreous, and its sharp point will be found to have no opening, and therefore impermeable. The *open* canal in which it rests passes a short distance forward, but not to the lens, being limited to the posterior third of the vitreous. This conical process is occasionally found rounded, or flattened, or distorted; and sometimes turned off to one side and depressed. The examination of even a dozen still-born fœtuses of the sixth and seventh months will show these variations.

This conical process becomes thinner and thinner, and finally disappears. The retina about the disc flattens off, and the normal permanent condition is reached.

This process of obliteration may often progress unequally in the two eyes; one eye showing a much more rapid disappearance of these structures than the other.

At almost any stage this process of obliteration may be checked, and there will remain through life either a more or less characteristic representation of these embryonic structures, or at least some vestige of them. These persistent remains vary widely. They range from the practically perfect survival of this vascular system as it existed in the fœtal eye, as we see in the case reported by Tangeman (147), through a long series of very greatly diversified, and more or less typical cases, down to the most atypical and rudimentary forms, that have not hitherto been grouped under this head, these forms including the first sixty of the following described cases.

ANATOMICAL DATA--The material for the minuter study of these changes is very meager. Only a chance specimen here and there has afforded an opportunity for microscopical examination. From embryological studies, supplemented by our ophthalmoscopic examinations, have we derived the bulk of our knowledge of these interesting conditions. Still the few sections that have been made have rendered some points more clear.

The proximal, or optic disc, end of the vessel is well illustrated by Manz (a). Among several examples of anencephalus that he had the opportunity of studying, was one that had reached full term; the others being of earlier stages. The posterior segment of one of these eyes is presented in Fig. 6 of Pl. 12. This shows clearly the thickened extremity of the nerve spreading out for some distance to each side; a true optic *disc* not yet differentiated. From its center projects forward the rudiment of the hyaloid. This pierces the retina through a small round opening, with sharply marked edges. The retina can be readily raised from the underlying structures, as is shown in the cut. The base of the artery presents a pyramidal structure, buried in the end of the nerve. This base is well shown in Fig. 3 of Pl. 1. This pyramid has upon its outer surface a covering of pavement epithelium, the cells of which are irregular, with large round nuclei; and are of nearly uniform size, except where the protoplasm of adjoining cells at some points seems to be fused together, and the demarcation lines lost. Within the pyramid is a rich cellular net-work of branching cells and long fine processes, shown at the lower portion of the figure where the outer layer is torn away. This cellular net-work also spins a rich plexus around the central artery. There seems little doubt but that this pyramid forms a highly developed lymph space. After loosely piercing the retina, the pyramid is truncated sharply, and ends at the level of the free surface of the retina. The vessel then passes free into the vitreous. The abnormal enlarging, thickening, and persistence of such a pyramidal base, will render intelligible the origin of such clumps as we will find in many of the following cases. Of these as marked examples as any are the two profiles we give in Plate 12, Dimmer's case (55), Fig. 4, and Debierre's case (67) Fig. 9. In group D numerous other examples are given in great variety.

The lateral expansion of the nerve head, so well shown in Manz's case, as noted above, Pl. 12, Fig. 6, will also probably explain the persistence of band-like expansions such as we find in Guene's case (54), and particularly well marked in Dimmer's case (55-6), illustrated on Plate 6, Figs. 1 and 2.

The *artery* itself is shown in Pl. 1, Fig. 3 (Manz's case). It is surrounded by a rather strong adventitia; the neighboring vitreous is somewhat condensed, and is particularly rich in cellular elements. The arterial coating is rather thick, showing quite clearly its cellular structure, with the nuclei nearly all lying in a longitudinal direction. In addition it contains so many small cellular elements, that we may well regard it as a perivascular lymph sheath. The vessel had a diameter of .05 mm. It is shown still further magnified in Fig. 6, Pl. 1 (from Vassaux's case, 135). The entire strand has a diameter of .17 mm. at either extremity, and somewhat less in the center of the vitreous. The outer sheath is finely striated both in a transverse and in a longitudinal direction; its outermost layer being composed of delicate wavy fibrillæ. Its inner face (shown in the figure where the sheath is torn apart) presents numerous ovoid, flattened nuclei, lying one close to the other, the surrounding cells with contours very difficult to make out. The entire appearance like an epithelial (endothelial) lining.

The intermediate space is occupied by a liquid (coagulated by the reagents, and colored pale rose by the straining material, carmine) in which the high powers show a delicate fibrillar net-work. In this space are found two varieties of cells: the one rounded, with or without a nucleus, and resembling a leucocyte or embryonic cell; the other with a round nucleus, and two or three wavy processes, and resembling a connective tissue cell. There are no traces of blood corpuscles. Some of the fibrillae can be traced across, joining the sheath and the adventitia of the artery.

The artery has a diameter of .08 mm. at either extremity, and .04 mm. at the center. It is surrounded by a delicate, diaphanous adventitia, with longitudinal fibrillæ; within this the muscular coat, in two layers, one circular and the other longitudinal; within this the nucleated intima. Within the lumen were found both red and white blood corpuscles.

Beyond being a little condensed along the sheath of the vessel, the vitreous is normal in its central portions. But in the peripheral portions adjacent to the retina, were found numerous tortuous granular filaments, in some of which were found a central cavity containing broken down blood corpuscles. These were no doubt remains of the early provisional branches that we have seen were given off from the hyaloid artery to supply the posterior portions of the vitreous.

In Brailey's case (140) the artery was merely a tough, white cord, consisting of indistinct fibrous tissue, longitudinally arranged. Running through its axis was a more marked band of fibers, in which the fibrillæ were much more distinct, and among which were found a few scattered pigment granules.

The presence of a wider canal, the canal of Cloquet, affording passage for these structures, is settled affirmatively by the researches of Stilling, and by the case of Manz (180) illustrated on Pl. 12, Fig. 7. This canal is also shown in Holmes's case (190), illustrated on Pl. 11, Fig. 1. These examples show this canal to have a diameter of 1 to 2 mm., terminating usually with a funnel-like expansion at either extremity, at the disc and at the posterior pole of the lens. The greatest diameter of the envelope of the hyaloid artery in Vassaux's case was .17 mm.

In some of the cases described below, just what share is taken by the artery proper, and what by this canal of Cloquet, is sometimes difficult to exactly determine. In group L, I have endeavored to include those cases in which this canal alone seems to be concerned.

The artery usually remains single until it reaches the posterior pole of the lens; but in Manz's case it divides into two branches soon after leaving the nerve. In quite a number of the cases described there are indications of a division during its course through the vitreous; and in Tangeman's case (147) the vessel divides into two branches soon after entering the vitreous, and each of these two again divides when near the lens. (Pl. 12, Fig. 8).

The anterior extremity of the artery usually passes direct to the posterior pole, and at once breaks up into the branches spreading over the posterior surface. In Haab's case (149), illustrated on Pl. 12, Fig. 5, the eye, from a case of hydrophthalmus congenitus, presented numerous pathological changes in the anterior segment. The vitreous chamber was closed anteriorly by a flattened plate composed of suspensory ligament, capsules, and the remnants of the shrunken lens. Into this plate (illustrated on Pl. 1, Fig. 2), the remnant of the hyaloid was attached with an abrupt bend ; but this angular distortion may have been one of the results of the pathological changes here.

The condition of the vessels upon the posterior face of the lens is not satisfactorily illustrated by the anatomical material at hand. In Vassaux's case (Pl. 1, Fig. 1) the vessels take very tortuous courses. In Haab's case (Pl. 1, Fig. 2) these vessels seem to have become inclosed in the shrunken plate, and are there indicated at several points in cross sections. In Gardiner's case (148) the little vessels seem to take very tortuous courses. But in the other cases described, and particularly in the cases I have seen (Pl. 12, Fig. 1 and 2) the remnants of the vessels seem to uniformly pass *straight* from the center to the periphery ; when dividing, branching dichotomously at very acute angles. It is probable that the variation from this plan in the cases of Vassaux and Haab is due to pathological disturbances. The original figure published by Kölliker, shows these vessels with an arrangement very similar to the persistent remains in my case (179) Pl. 12, Fig. 2 (L).

Other conditions observed are not necessary associates with the rudimentary hyaloid. In Vassaux's case the posterior portion of the lens was covered with a dense plate of fibrillar tissue with numerous fusiform cells (shown in Fig. 5, Pl. 1). This, with the vessels spread upon it, had led to the mistaken diagnosis of glioma, the enucleation, and the fortunate opportunity for microscopic examination. In this case the ciliary processes are greatly elongated and adherent to the posterior surface of the lens, toward the equator. This condition is present in Haab's case (Pl. 12, Fig. 5). In Brailey's case (140) the iris and ciliary bodies were adherent to the edge of the lens.

In Vassaux's case he calls attention to an anomalous condition in the retina, which he states he had never seen in normal sections. This is a layer or row of fusiform elements occupying the inner zone of the external granule layer (shown on Pl. 1, Fig. 4, F). This occupies the position of Henle's "outer fibrous layer," which in the normal human retina at certain points forms a band here of delicate fibres, without granules. Manz calls attention to the uniform occurrence in all the anencephalic monsters he examined of an unusual thickness of the outer granule layer. Perhaps in the human retina such a band of fusiform fibres is one of the stages of development always passed through. My specimens are not decisive, and I do not find the point cleared up in the literature at my disposal. At any rate, such fusiform elements I find scattered through the external granule layer in sections of the frog's retina ; and in Mueller's beautiful plates ("Ueber die Stammesentwicklung des Sehorgans der Wirbelthiere," Leipzig, 1875), I find just such a row of similar fusiform elements occupying this position in the retina of Petromyzon. If this condition, so inexplicable to Vassaux, is not a customary stage of development, it shows an interesting reversion to a primitive type.

In certain cases pathological conditions of various kinds are associated, but whether there be any direct connection is difficult to determine conclusively. In Vanlair's case (110) the hyaloid artery pushed forward through a gelatinous tumor, probably a glioma, and a mass of blood-vessels, with which it was connected. V. thinks this vascular tumor was an outgrowth from the artery ; but there is no proof, on the other hand, that the vessel itself was not a new growth, developed with the other vessels of the tumor.

In Nettleship's case (139) there were numerous pathological changes in the intra-ocular structures; a granular vitreous, and "thickened fibrous layer spreading out from the base of the artery over the retina," being the most important. N. is of the opinion that all these changes had taken their origin from degenerative changes that the presence of the hyaloid remains had initiated. While positive proof is from the nature of the question difficult to present; still there seems some warrant for holding the opinion that this was probably the fact.

In Brailey's case (140) a completely detached retina was wrapped about the hyaloid cord. Probably there existed no causal connection here, merely a coincidence.

CLINICAL DATA—An industrious search through the literature reveals a clinical material very rich as compared with the scanty anatomical material. It affords us sufficient data for a very satisfactory classification, and the intelligent study of the numerous forms under which we find this anomaly present itself.

A summary of the reported cases, tabulated either chronologically or alphabetically, would prove monotonous and least instructive. We find that the cases naturally arrange themselves into a dozen groups, the characteristics of which afford sufficient points for convenient classification. To be sure, while the type forms of the various groups are sharply differentiated from each other, intermediate forms so bind together the various groups that practically a fairly complete and continuous chain is formed. This makes difficult the proper placing of some of the intermediate forms, but does not essentially impair the value and convenience of the grouped arrangement.

We may recognize the following fairly well marked groups. Of these, groups E, F, G, H, I, and L, comprise the ordinary, well recognized forms ; the other groups comprise the more aberrant, atypical and less clearly recognized varieties:

A—Shreds of tissue on the optic disc.

B—Membranes on the disc.

C—Cystic remains on the disc.

D—Masses of connective tissue on the disc.

E—Rudimentary strand attached to the disc.

F—Strand attached to the disc, and a vestige also at the posterio
    surface of the lens.

G—Strand passing from the disc to the lens.

H—Similar strand containing blood (sub-group).

I—Strand attached to the lens alone.

J—Posterior capsular cataract.

K—Striæ on the posterior lens-capsule.

L—Persistent canal (without any remnant of the vessel).

These groups we will take up in order; giving in each division a concise abstract of all the reported cases properly coming under each of these headings.

To one who has given no particular thought to this anomaly, it may seem somewhat of a revelation to find here nearly two hundred cases described. The general impression has been that this congenital anomaly was of extremely rare occurrence, an ophthalmoscopic curiosity almost; but the series of cases here collected shows that this is by no means the fact; that this anomaly can no longer be considered as in any sense an exceptional rarity. This is moreover borne out by the fact that several individual observers report each a number of cases, as many even as eight in one instance, that of Reuss. This fact is the more gratifying to me, as otherwise I would have felt considerable diffidence in presenting the large number of cases that have come under my own observation. My unusual luck in this respect is one of the results of many thousand careful ophthalmoscopic examinations made during the last ten years, utilizing for this purpose all sorts of material, clinic cases of every kind, medical students, school children, inmates of infirmary, orphan asylum, work-house, etc. All this material has been patiently gone over day by day, as opportunities offered. The direct method has been employed, and always a keen watch kept for all sorts of variations from the normal, however slight. By work of this sort, stretching over years, I find that the material in my hands for a comprehensive survey of the congenital anomalies of the eye is becoming of very satisfactory extent; in connection with the extremely rich literature that has been appearing of late years.

The clinical recognition of this anomaly dates of course from a period subsequent to the discovery of the ophthalmoscope. Still there is a hint that our keen old observer, Mackenzie, had actually detected a case by oblique illumination, without, however, appreciating what he saw. In this case (160) he detected through the dilated pupil, deep behind the lens, an opaque spot which moved up and down on moving the eye. Although he regarded this as hyaloiditis (?), the fact that there was present a characteristic posterior capsular cataract, with radiating striæ, makes it very probable that this was, in reality, the anterior detached and floating end of the persistent hyaloid remain, which had formerly been attached at the point indicated by the cataract.

In 1856, H. Müller reports the frequent occurrence in the ox's eye of a short process projecting from the optic disc into the vitreous. He notes the observation of a similar process in a human eye he was examining microscopically, and made the prediction that such a remnant of the hyaloid vessel would no doubt soon be detected by the ophthalmoscope. In the following year, Meissner reports a case (70) where he had discovered such a process in the eye of an old man, upon postmortem examination.

Müller's prediction did not remain long unverified. In the following year, 1857, Zehender was the first to detect this anomaly upon ophthalmoscopic examination. This case (144) observed in the Rostock clinic was not, however, reported until 1863, when it was called out by the report by Saemisch (119) of a case observed ophthalmoscopically (the first case *reported*).

Wallman, in 1858, had reported another case (117) observed postmortem.

Saemisch and Zehender's cases were followed in the same year by two other cases reported by Zehender; one of which had been observed by Dr. Toussaint, and the other by Liebreich.

In 1865, Stör adds another case (123), and in the same year Wecker reports the first case (121) observed in France.

In 1866, Laurence reports the first case (115) observed in England.

It was not until 1873 that Kipp reports the first case (109) from America. During this first ten years the reports were few and scattering, and not very complete or satisfactory; since then the literature has become quite extensive, and our knowledge of this anomaly of the eye is among the most satisfactory in the entire long list.

GROUP A—SHREDS OF TISSUE ON THE DISC.

Cases come under observation occasionally, and by no means rarely, in which we find upon the optic disc little irregular shreds or bands of connective tissue. These are glistening white, at times almost transparent, only faintly softening the vessels that may run beneath them ; and again are thicker and more opaque, either completely hiding the vessels beneath, or only allowing them to shimmer faintly through. After I had observed and drawn two or three of these cases, it occurred to me, lacking any other probable explanation, that these were remnants of the adventitia of the fœtal hyaloid artery which had remained as the last vestige persisting of this structure. At that time I thought that this explanation of these shreads had not been suggested by any other observer, but I find that in 1876, Noyes, in reporting his series of refraction cases, mentions having seen these little bands in five instances, and gave as a probable explanation, that " it sometimes looked like an obliterated vessel." In the strict sense, these are not " obliterated vessels " as we see them in embolus, etc., and this he could not have meant literally ; but to my mind they *are* remnants of an obliterated vessel, the hyaloid. Ulrich, in 1882, reports one case among three of persistent hyaloid remains. where only a delicate white film covered the center of the disc ; and seems to tacitly group this under the same head.

These delicate shreds have, however, been regarded in quite a different light by certain other observers.

Schmidt-Rimpler, in 1877, and following him Schaumberg, in 1882, report a series of analogous cases as instances of " double-contoured nerve fibres " upon the disc. This is most manifestly erroneous, as any one carefully studying an example of this sort will at once see. The strongest disproof of their view is furnished by their own cases and drawings. It so happens that in at least four of their seven cases the narrow band runs in a direction at a right angle to and thus *squarely across* the course of the nerve fibres. So that in these cases at least this view is untenable. When we consider how extremely rare is the occurrence of the double-contoured fibres upon the disc itself, it seems extremely improbable that Schaumberg could have *five* examples to quote in a graduation thesis. Moreover his figures are the rudest of diagramatic cuts ; and from their study alone, independent of his descriptions, the very last idea that would be conveyed would be that they were intended to represent areas of double-contoured nerve fibres.

Berger, in 1882, in describing three such cases, is inclined to regard them as due to a mild, diffuse neuro-retinitis with exudation. But his own cases, and as it happens, all the other cases reported, almost without exception, have *normal* vision ; either without any glass or with the proper correcting glass. It is too much of a strain on the theory of probabilities to assume that in more than a dozen cases we could have an exudative neuro-retinitis, in each case just nicely stopping short before affecting vision.

That these shreds are congenital, there seems really no question; that they form the most rudimentary, most atypical and least characteristic form of persistence of some part of the fœtal hyaloid system is rendered almost as certain, from lack of any other tenable explanation.

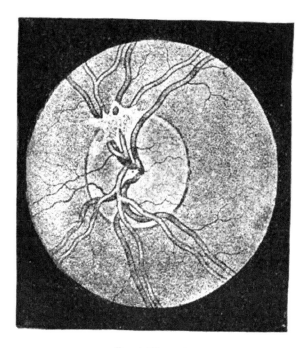

FIG. 1 (NOYES).

This figure, taken from Noyes' new work on Diseases of the Eye, illustrates very nicely one of these little shreds or small membranes; although usually the remnants occupy a more central position on the disc.

Plate II gives six good examples of this group. They must be quite common. I have seem eight or ten, Dr. Randall has seen about as many, Dr. Noyes has seen five or more, Schaumberg describes five, etc. I have no doubt that many observers can now recall cases of this character.

NOYES—

(1–5) This author, in making a report at the Fifth International Ophthalmological Congress upon over one thousand recorded cases of ametropia, mentions incidentally that among these he had seen five cases in which there was a band of connective tissue running across the disc. This was sometimes of a glistening whiteness, sometimes semi-transparent. " It sometimes

looked like an obliterated vessel, and this would be the probable explanation of almost all of them."

HIRSCHBERG (b)—

(6) Workman, aet. 42. Reads Sn. 1½. Has M. of 1 D. In one eye there
presented a peculiar flecking (?) of the optic disc. One large, sharply outlined, bluish-white fleck partially covered the lower nasal artery and reached
inwards to the margin of the physiological cup. The other encircled the
lower nasal vein and reached out a short distance (.15 mm.) upon the retina.
Papilla and retina normal in other respects.

SCHMIDT-RIMPLER—

Describes and figures two cases of small shreds on the disc. They were irregular, punctate and striated, were intensely white and glistening, and hid
the vessels they passed across.

(7) Case 1. Right eye. A long triangular shred, shaped like a shark's tooth,
on the inner half of the disc, running vertically. It hid the inferior temporal vein, and the three branches of the superior temporal artery.

(8) Case 2. Right eye. A narrow shred, shaped like an incisor tooth, ran from
the center of the disc to its upper border. It was just to the inner side of
the main vessel, and hid, in crossing, the superior temporal artery and
vein.

SCHAUMBERG—

(9) Heinrich W——. Eyes emmetropic and V=1. In the L. eye a vertical
band, shaped something like a slender foot and ankle, crossed the temporal
half of the disc. It covered an arterial branch above, crossed a vein at
its center, and covered two smaller arterial branches below.

(10) In the R. eye a triangular film covered a sector comprising almost one-sixth
of the disc, directly outward. It covered an artery and a vein.

(11) Katharina W——. (Aet. 13). Myopia of 16, with old corneal opacities.
V=⅔. L. eye showed a narrow, well-marked band upon the disc. It ran
along the temporal side, near the border. Above and below made a sharp
turn inwards. In its course it crossed all the vessels of the disc, except a
small artery and vein which ran directly to nasal side.

BERGER, E. (a)—

(12) Franz S——. Aet. 22. Treated for catarrhal conjunctivitis. The ophthalmoscope showed a white glistening band beginning on the upper half of the
disc to the outer side, running upward and outward, passing over for about
a half disc-diameter upon the retina, and ending with a broadened, frayed
extremity. At the outer edge of the disc a similar band begins, and runs
upward and inward, passing onto the retina above. The bands are striated
in the direction of their length. The bands cross at an acute angle, and
their fibres seem to interlace. Several of the superior vessels pass under
these bands. The fundus is otherwise perfectly normal and V=⅔⅛. Patient
had never had any previous eye trouble.

(13) Gustav B——. Aet. 10 Patient in the Skin Clinic, Vienna. Eyes examined with the ophthalmoscope. The right showed two white glistening
bands on the disc; a smaller one in the lower half, between the inferior
artery and vein; the larger one began just to the outer side of the central
vessels, and passed in an oblique direction outward to be lost a short dis-

tance out on the retina. Fundus normal; $V=\frac{2.0}{1.8}$; and never any eye trouble.

(14) Anton M——. Aet. 37. Patient came on account of asthenopia. Had hypermetropia of low degree. With the ophthalmoscope the left eye showed the central vessels to be strongly bordered by white, delicate bands. On the lower half of the disc began a bright, silvery band, delicately striated. It passed horizontally inward until it crossed the disc border, then curved downward, and ended with a broadened frayed end in the lower-inner quadrant of the retina. Two vessels, an artery and vein, passed through this strand. Fundus normal. $V=\frac{2.0}{1.8}$ with correcting + glass. Had never had any eye trouble, except the asthenopia.

ULRICH—

(15) Boy of fifteen years. Had retinitis pigmentosa. In one eye the center of the disc was covered by a small, white film, which hid the point of exit of the vessels.

A colleague of U.'s stated to him that he had noticed a similar condition in one of his cases of retinitis pigmentosa.

LITTLE—

(16) Miss W——. Aet. 20. (Same case as 134.) Ophthalmoscope showed in the left eye some slight traces of the adventitia of the hyaloid artery close to the disc. $V=\frac{15}{100}$. With +60c 90° $V=\frac{2.0}{1.8}$.

(If these shreds were in the vitreous, of course this case belongs to a subsequent group).

DEBECK—(Plate II, Fig. 1).

(17) Miss Aggie B——. Aet. 15. Came on account of asthenopia, and with a slight blepharitis marginalis. With convex 30 s. $V = \frac{2.0}{1.8}$. In her R. eye the ophthalmoscope showed a delicate white, semi-transparent film covering the point of exit of the vessels. The vessels shimmer faintly through it. Its diameter is a trifle less than one-third that of the disc, and its edges are quite sharply defined, marking it off from the pink disc.

In her left eye was found a more marked and prominent clump of darker tissue.

(See case 50)

—— —(Plate II, Fig. 4).

(18) Anna H——. Aet. 19. Patient came complaining of poor vision. Had simp. hyp. ast. $V = \frac{20}{100}$, and with + 2.25c 90° was improved to $\frac{2.0}{1.8}$. The ophthalmoscope showed on the right disc a delicate white membrane, and bands of tissue. A small rhomboidal patch covered the lower-inner periphery of the disc, slightly encroaching upon the adjoining retina. It partially covered the lower nasal artery and vein. It sent up a narrow branching band, one arm passing toward the upper inner border, crossing a vein, and the other passing in toward the point of exit of the vessels.

—— —(Plate II, Fig. 5).

(19) Carrie G——. Aet. 13. Patient came for refractive trouble. Had H. of 4 D.; with $V = \frac{2.0}{1.8}$.

Upon the disc in the right eye were strands of white glistening connective tissue. One at the center partially veiled the point of exit of the arterial branches; from it then passed a broad strand downward and inward obscur-

ing the inferior nasal artery; from the end of this there passed a broad vertical strand near the inner border of the disc, which veiled one of the
smaller veins above. This was connected with the central strand by two
fine transverse bands on the upper half of the disc.

——— —(Plate II, Fig. 6).

(20) Thomas O'H——. Aet. 60. This patient came on account of failing vision
in his *left* eye; which, on examination, proved to be due to incipient, senile,
nuclear cataract. His vision had always been most exceptionally good. His
right also showed a slightly hazy nucleus, but not enough to prevent obtain-
ing a perfectly clear ophthalmoscopic picture. V was still $\frac{20}{8}$ or $\frac{20}{8}$ — in the
right.

At the center of the disc in this right eye was a white glistening clump of
tissue which entirely hid the point of exit of the arteries, and partially obscured the point of entrance of the veins. From this central portion a narrow band passed a short distance downward upon the disc, close to the artery,
and a narrow point passed upward covering the point of departure of one of
the smaller arteries. From the nasal side of this clump a narrow strand
passed inward across the nasal half of the disc to the disc margin, and then
turned sharply upward, slightly broadening, and passed along the disc margin nearly to its upper border. This band lay about half upon the disc
border, and half upon the adjacent retina, and hid in crossing the same
small artery mentioned above.

——— —(Plate II, Fig. 2).

(21) Mrs. Ellen M——. Aet. 35. Patient came complaining of asthenopia.
This was attributed to prolonged lactation. In the *right* eye V was considerably impaired, and a mild neuritis was detected on examination. This
gradually cleared up and V rose to $\frac{20}{30}$ after weaning the child, and being
placed on strychnia. The *left* eye remained throughout perfectly normal,
and V was at all times $\frac{20}{8}$ sharp.

The ophthalmoscope showed in this *left* eye a white clump hiding the point
of exit of the vessels. Just to the nasal side of this passed out a strong
band hiding the inner ends of a small artery and vein. This band sent one
division downward along and very slightly covering the main inferior artery,
and terminating in a narrow thread passing inward to be attached to a distinct
vertical band. The other division passed directly to the nasal margin to join
the same vertical band above. This distinct vertical band ran along the
nasal margin of the disc, and some distance down upon the retina below.
It is narrow at the center and broadens out in a fan shape above and below.
A large vein above and a small vein below, with two small arterial branches
are covered by this band, and shimmer faintly through it. This band has
the very faintest bluish gleam.

——— — —(Plate II, Fig. 3).

(22) Hester J——. Aet. 39 (colored). Patient came complaining of asthenopia,
due to a slight hypermetropia. V with + 36 was $\frac{20}{8}$ sharp.

Ophthalmoscope showed in the *right* eye the center of the disc covered by a
glistening white, pear-shaped membrane, completely hiding the exit of the
vessels. Upon the first glimpse by the indirect method, this seemed like a
physiological cup, but the direct examination showed the porus filled up by
this tissue to the level of the vessels, which sunk sharply into it. From this

clump a band passed upward, hiding the main artery and the beginning of its three branches, and partially obscuring the main vein. From the upper end of this band, a very distinct, arrow-shaped band passes transversely across the upper part of the disc nearly to the margin, completely hiding the vein and arteries which it crosses. This band is the thickest and most opaque that was seen in any of these cases.

GROUP B—MEMBRANES ON THE DISC.

A small series of cases have been reported in which a glistening white membrane was found covering the disc to a greater or less extent, and in most instances, encroaching somewhat upon the adjoining retina. This membrane usually presents considerable thickness, and either completely hides the vessels, or obscures them to a very marked degree.

In my view these membranes are also remnants of the adventitia of the embryonic hyaloid vessel. This explanation has been advanced by no other observer; but, so far as I can find, no other observer has advanced *any* valid explanation. If this view is tenable for the previous group, then it must hold here, for these two groups really form a continuous series without any sharp dividing line. Their separation is arbitrary, and only for convenience of classification and description.

That these membranes are congenital there seems to be no question whatever.

Plate III gives six examples of this group. This view of the genesis of these membranes is strengthened by the fact that a few of the cases of undoubted hyaloid remains are attached at the disc by a membranous-like expansion which, viewed alone, is closely identical in position and appearance with the membranes figured on Plate III.

The membranous tube that forms the canal of Cloquet, as a rule terminates at the disc in a funnel-shaped base or foot, that is usually a trifle larger than the disc. Were all the hyaloid system to become obliterated except this base, and this to flatten down; we would no doubt have just such a remain as is described in most of these cases, and such as is figured by Fuchs. (Plate III, Fig. 6).

Or were we to have this base persist as a cystic, bladder-like remnant lying upon the disc, as is described in some cases in Group C, and then suppose this to burst and collapse, we can readily imagine that the sunken walls becoming adherent to the base or disc would give us such a picture as that of Fuchs.

SCHAUMBERG—

(23) George S——. (Aet. 24). Hm. of .25, with V= 1 in R. eye. The ophthalmoscope shows a quadrilateral membrane covering the outer segment of the disc; embracing about one quarter of the periphery and reaching in not

quite to the point of entrance of the vessels. It is dense, glistening white, and covers an artery and a vein.

—————— —(Plate III, Fig. 4).

(24) Johann M——. (Aet. 43). Right eye V = 1. A cruciform membrane covers and hides the point of exit of the vessels. It sends one arm upward and slightly outward; one to inner side and slightly upward; one downward and inward, and one downward and outward. The membrane is dense and white, covering the inner ends of all the vessels of the disc except a small vein and an arterial branch running directly outward.

HIRSCHBERG (*b*)—

(25) Mrs. S——. Aet. 46. The eyes were emmetropic and vision normal. In the left eye the ophthalmoscope showed a hand-shaped, sharply outlined, white membrane upon the disc. It was about ½ the disc diameter in height and ⅓ the disc diameter in width; and completely hid the vessels beneath it. The part of the disc not covered was normal in texture and appearance.

FUCHS—(Plate III, Fig. 6).

(26) Man of 26 yrs. V. and refracton both normal.

In the R. eye the ophthalmoscope shows the disc to be nearly covered by an intensely white, glistening, semi-transparent membrane, evidently composed of ordinary connective tissue. It has a rough kidney shape, its longer diameter being vertical. To the outer side not quite a third of the disc is left exposed; to the inner side a minute portion. Above and below it reaches out upon the retina for a short distance beyond the disc border. It covers all the vessels of the disc and is so thick that they shimmer through only with the greatest faintness. It lies closely adherent to the disc and vessels, giving no parallax on moving the head. The remainder of the eyeground is normal.

(27–28) This author has seen two other similar cases. In both the membrane was much more delicate and transparent, and the vessels showed through much more distinctly. V and refraction in both were normal.

LORING (*a*)—

(29) This author had seen one similar case. It consisted of a delicate but untransparent membrane, which covered the *entire* nerve-entrance, and extended out over the retinal vessels for some distance beyond the borders of the disc. It was evidently congenital; and vision was but slightly below the normal.

RANDALL—(Plate III, Fig. 2).

I am indebted to Dr. Randall for the additional data in this case and in cases 32, 33, 34, 36, 37, and 53·

(30) Mrs. Sarah S——. Aet. 39. Came on account of asthenopia. R —V = $\frac{20}{18}$; L — V = $\frac{20}{18}$. In the right eye the ophthalmoscope showed a glistening white quadrangular patch covering the lower nasal sector of the disc, comprising about ⅓ of its area. Its lower rounded angle encroached slightly upon the adjacent retina. Its upper pointed angle reached to the disc cup. It was rather thick, and almost completely hid two arterial and one venous branch covered by it.

(31) In the left eye was a very similar quadrate patch—lying, however, to the nasal side.

———— —(Plate III., Fig. 3).

(32) Minnie D——. Aet. 19. Had low H. R. eye $V = \frac{6}{7.5}$ with +1.5 D.; L. eye $V = \frac{3}{4}$ with +2.5.

Ophthalmoscope revealed a helmet-shaped membrane in the right eye, covering the upper-inner quadrant of the disc; and with its edge passing out a short distance upon the neighboring retina. It was of a brilliant gleaming white, and allowed the two arteries and the two veins that it covered to shimmer faintly through. No change in this fundus in five years, under observation. Macula normal.

(33) In the left eye a small band covered the lower vessels, near the margin of the disc.

———— —(Plate III, Fig. 5).

(34) Boy of 14 years. Came on account of poor vision.

In the left eye, which was amblyopic, the ophthalmoscope showed a thick, glistening white membrane covering the central portion and the entire outer half of the disc. Its outer margin was sharp, and coincided with that of the disc. The point of exit of the vessels and their courses while under this membrane were entirely hid.

DeBeck—(Plate III, Fig. 1).

(35) Mrs. Mary H——. Aet. 37. Came with her daughter, who had optic neuritis.

Mere casual ophthalmoscopic examination showed in the left eye a delicate membrane covering the center and lower-inner quadrant of the disc. It covered almost $\frac{1}{2}$ the area of the disc. At the center it partially veiled all the vessels, and further out covered the lower vein and its two branches. It was not so dense but that it allowed these veins to faintly shimmer through. It partially spread over onto the retina for a short distance beyond the edge of the disc. This membrane showed a very distinct striated fibrillation. It gave a faint bluish or grayish reflex.

GROUP C—CYSTIC REMAINS ON THE DISC.

A small group of cases have been reported where the remnant of the hyaloid vessel was found occurring as a cystic expansion upon the disc. These show rounded or oval. They have a characteristic translucent tint, very suggestive of fluid contents; and are pearly gray, or steel bluish in color. I have seen no example of the larger forms; but from the descriptions, they seem to present these same appearances, even more characteristically.

This group, though limited, forms an exceptionally complete series. We have first a few cases of little rounded cysts upon the disc. These aberrant forms, like the two figured by Randall, do not at first impress one as belonging to this category at all, and the first case I saw (Fig. 3, on Plate 4), did not suggest this connection to me. But Kollock's case is one which shows that the stalk upon which the cyst rests springs from the physiological cup, and my more recent case (Fig. 5, Plate 4) shows this even more clearly.. Then comes the third variety, the larger rounded cysts which cover the disc and have a knob-like head projecting forward, as in the cases resembling cysticerci reported by Carter and Goldzieher. Then come the elongated flask-shaped cysts as reported by Holmes and Rocliffe. In the one case this narrowed to a "neck" and knob-like "head," lying just back of the posterior surface of the lens. In the other this terminated anteriorly in several fine fibrillæ which were attached to the posterior lens-capsule. These cases unmistakably join this special group to the general group of persistent hyaloid remains. The genesis of these cases is even made more clear by two additional cases ; in Königstein's case (46) a little ampulla-like dilatation, containing blood, rested on the disc, and from this the strand projected forward into the vitreous; in my case (Fig. 6, Plate 4) a little knob-like expansion was found at the bifurcation of the central artery. It was connected with the vessels, and contained blood, but it is easy to see that if this communication were cut off it would remain as a little gray cyst.

Plate 4 shows five examples of the smaller forms. Such little cystic remains can not be very rare, if carefully searched for. They are not at all conspicuous by the indirect method of examination, and may often be overlooked.

I have lately seen an additional case, an example even smaller than that of Dr. Randall's on Pl. IV, Fig. 1. This makes three I have seen; Dr. Randall has seen five or six.

In this connection a possible explanation for the previous group has been ventured with diffidence. The collapse of such a cysticercus-like cyst would leave its adherent walls showing much such a membrane as is figured in Plate III, Fig. 6.

Compare also case 52, where a small, semi-detached vesicle floats in front of the disc.

RANDALL—(Plate IV, Fig. 1)

(36) Mary D——. Aet. 13. Came on account of asthenopia. $V = \frac{20}{28}$. The ophthalmoscope showed in the right eye a minute round cyst, of the pearly gray tint. It was about twice the size of the primary retinal vessels; was situated exactly upon the nasal disc border, directly inward in the horizontal axis; and rested closely upon a minute retinal vessel, with which it gave no parallax.

RANDALL—(Plate IV, Fig. 2).

(37) Emma S——. Aet. 15. Came on account of asthenopia, due to H. As. of low degree. In the left eye the ophthalmoscope revealed a little oval cyst, whose diameter was nearly $\frac{1}{4}$ that of the disc. It was, like all the forms,

of a pearly gray tint, with a sort of translucent shimmer. It rested upon the nasal half of the disc, in its horizontal diameter, resting closely upon a retinal vein, with which it gave no parallactic movement.

(Dr. Randall writes me that he has seen three or four additional cases of these little cystic remains upon the disc—and that he has no doubt of their being remnants of the hyaloid artery).

DeBeck—(Plate IV, Fig. 3).

(38) Annie T——. Aet. 28—colored. Patient came for a slight conjunctivitis. $V = \frac{28}{28}$.

In the right eye the ophthalmoscope revealed a small cyst upon the disc. It was about three times the diameter of the main artery, and perfectly round. Its place was about half way between the center of the disc and its lower-inner border; resting upon the fork of the lower nasal vein, and in an elbow formed by the lower nasal artery. It had a translucent, yellowish-gray tint, with darker borders, and a glistening reflex from its most prominent surface. A delicate film of connective tissue ran from it to the central spot of the disc, very faintly veiling the vein upon which it rested.

Kollock—(Plate IV, Fig. 4).

(39) Mrs. M——. (Adult—married). Complained of poor vision in R. eye. When first seen vitreous was cloudy, containing some floating bodies; and the disc was blurred.

No specific history; had no children. Iodide of potassium was given in 10 gr. doses three times a day, and increased. Under this the vitreous cleared up.

Later examination showed a bubble-like protuberance covering the point of exit of the retinal vessels.

This was bright and glistening; but not transparent—general translucency existing with no distinct darker center. The vessels were indistinctly visible through its edges. Later on a short but distinct pedicle was made out attaching it to the floor of the physiological cup, at the point where the vessels entered and emerged. V had become normal $\frac{20}{20}$; and the media perfectly clear—with the exception of a large floating body, very annoying to the patient.

Although there had been mild neuritis (papillitis) this growth is not pathological, and it is no doubt the cystic stump remaining of the former hyaloid artery.

DeBeck—(Plate IV, Fig. 5).

(40) Miss Lillie K——. Aet. 19 (school teacher). Came for refractive trouble, with marginal blepharitis. V in right eye = $\frac{20}{30}$, and with + 1.00c 90° = $\frac{20}{20}$.

In the right eye there sprang from the central part of the disc just at the division of the artery a short and stout cylindrical column, rounded but slightly flattened from side to side. It was a trifle thicker than even the largest vein. At its extremity it is expanded into a round, cyst-like body, fully twice the diameter of the stalk. The pedicle is dark gray, the cystic end is paler, translucent and shining. It requires 4 or 5 D. to focus clearly upon it, and it gives a decided parallax with the vessels beneath. Whether it contains fluid or not can not be certainly answered—my opinion is that it does.

CARTER (a)—

(41) This author refers very briefly to a case which he had seen. In this instance the hyaloid remains had become expanded into a delicate pellucid cyst, which was attached to the optic disc. It presented a very deceptive resemblance to a cysticercus. He regarded it as a remnant of the hyaloid vessel.

GOLDZIEHER—

(42) Man, adult, had poor vision. Right eye presented choroiditis and commencing atrophy of the optic nerve. The left eye presented an excavation of the nerve; detachment of the retina, and in front of the nerve a pear-shaped, bluish, shimmering, cyst-like body. This narrowed to a short, thick neck, which terminated in a rounded knob. This neck and head moved slowly about. So deceptive was the resemblance to a cysticercus, that even so keen an observer as G. was led to make this diagnosis. However, according to Szili (Jahresbericht über Ophthalmologie, Bd. 15, 1884, p. 587), this case was at about the same time examined by several other careful observers, and they were unanimous in deciding this to be a remnant of the hyaloid artery; accompanied by coloboma of the nerve and choroid.

HOLMES (E. L.)—

(43) E. J. W——. Aet. 17. Came on account of extreme amblyopia, which had always existed in the right eye. There was marked divergent strabismus; the iris was much darker than in the other eye (congenital); the pupil was sluggish in reaction, and only moderately dilatable by atropine; there was quite a large central scotoma; and peripheral vision was scarcely $\frac{8}{100}$.

The opthalmoscope revealed a very curious flask-shaped body covering the disc, and occupying the center of the vitreous. Its base was somewhat larger than the optic disc, covering its entire periphery. From this there projected forward the rounded body; this narrowed into a sort of neck, and terminated anteriorly in a knob-like rounded head, situated just back of the posterior pole of the lens. Its walls were of a brilliant white, and apparently it might contain fluid. It had no motion. Its resemblance to a cysticercus was very striking.

ROCLIFFE—

(44) Mark W——. Aet. 13. Came on account of having discovered that he was blind in the left eye.

R. was normal: L. no perception of light.

The ophthalmoscope showed a peculiar bottle-shaped formation covering the disc. It entirely hid the papilla, and the retinal vessels emerged from under the edges of its base. It passed forward through the vitreous nearly to the lens. At the narrowed neck-like portion it divided into two strands. These subdivide into several delicate fibrillæ, which are attached to the upper surface of the lens capsule.

From the upper portion of the retina several filmy opacities hang loosely down, and many others float freely in the vitreous.

Between the disc and macula is an oval patch of thinning of the choroid.

DEBECK—(Plate IV, Fig. 6).

(45) Albert G——. Aet. 37. Patient came on account of a complete paralysis of the third nerve in the left eye, and partial paresis of the third in the right

eye. No clear specific history, but he improved under large doses of the iodide.

The ophthalmoscope revealed a curious appearance in the right eye. Just in the angle formed by the central artery dividing into its two primary branches on the floor of the physiological cup, there was a little triangular protuberance slightly larger than the diameter of the artery. It was filled with arterial blood, and when the arterial pulsation was obtained by pressure, it was seen to pulsate very distinctly. V was still normal, and I could not regard this as an aneurismal dilation of the vessels, due to syphilitic weakening of their walls. Were its connection with the artery cut off, and its walls thinned and dilated, it would present exactly the appearance of the little cysts described above.

Its appearance and position leave no doubt in my mind of its being a minute rudiment of the hyaloid artery.

KÖNIGSTEIN—

(46) Young girl. Case presented to the Vienna Society of Physicians.

The ophthalmoscope revealed a white disc. At its outer edge was a small, ampulla-shaped, reddish body. From this a strand projected directly forward through the viteous. This was red in color, and consequently carried blood.

In the anterior part of the vitreous the red blood column ended, and the strand continued forward as a dark fiber. This narrowed rapidly; it carried a number of little knot-like swellings, and sent off numerous fine branches. To right and left of the strand was a delicate, veil-like sheath.

The ampulla-like base makes this case of interest here as suggesting the genesis of these little cysts, although the case really belongs in group E.

GROUP D—IRREGULAR CLUMPS OF TISSUE UPON THE DISC.

Quite a group of cases have been reported where the disc is more or less covered and hid by an irregular mass of connective tissue. This group presents the greatest variability, is the least sharply marked off of any, and forms the most general connecting link between the other groups. On the one side it shades into the first two groups, only differing from the bands and membranes by a greater thickness, and usually a darker color, as is shown in Figs. 1–4 on Plate 5. In some cases it affiliates with the group of cystic remains, as is shown in Hersing's case (Fig. 2 of Plate 7). Finally this clump may be the base of an undoubted hyaloid remain, which projects forward through the vitreous, as is shown in the cases of Remak (Plate 5, Figs. 5 and 6), and Reuss (Plate 7, Fig. 1). The cases of Becker and Dimmer also illustrate this. In fact, in the following groups we will find that in some of the typical and undoubted cases the persistent strand springs from a similar clump of tissue upon the disc.

The four cases figured in Plate 5 are fairly well marked examples of the less conspicuous forms, and examples of this and slighter grades must be extremely common. One does not engage in ophthalmoscopic work very long without becoming familiar with the frequent instances where these little gray or bluish strands obscure the exit of the vessels, or partially fill up the physiological cup, or border the vessels on the disc. Of course, these trifling remnants are hardly to be dignified by the title of congenital anomalies, but when at all marked, they merge into our group now under consideration.

What with these little gray bands, and the little glistening white shreds, and the small glistening white membranes, and the intermediate forms, these groups are all quite intimately bound together.

This group of cases comprise the forms that are most liable to be mistaken for pathological products, especially as the vision in a large proportion of these cases of extensive remains is found to be defective.

But the unchanging appearance of these cases when long observed; the absence of any previous eye affection; the stationary character of the defective vision, dating back to infancy, as well as the affiliations of the entire group, prove the congenital character of these cases, and that granted, their position is unquestionably among the hyaloid remains. Moreover, so many of them present a remnant passing forward into the vitreous—either a conical or club-shaped process, or a cord-like strand, or delicate fibrillæ.

Some of the cases summarized here, really belong to subsequent groups, but the interest attaching to the irregular remnants at the disc predominating over the other features, they are quoted here. Moreover, the other groups are unwieldy enough without them.

DeBeck—(Plate V, Fig. 1).

(47) Mrs. Louisa H——. Aet. 38. Came with slight conjunctivitis. Routine ophthalmoscopic examination revealed a clump of bluish gray tissue hiding the point of exit of the vessels. It thinned out above and below, veiling the vessels for a short distance. Only to the inner and the lower-outer edge was it sharply defined, and here the vessels disappeared adruptly. V was $\frac{7}{8}$.

Fundus perfectly normal otherwise.

———— —(Plate V, Fig. 2).

(48) Katie C——. Aet. 12. Patient came for refractive trouble. V = $\frac{7}{8}$. Hm. 1.00.

In the left eye the point of exit of the vessels is completely hidden by a thick, rectangular clump of connective tissue of a dark bluish-gray tint. Its upper and lower edges, where the vessels emerge, are softer and blend off gradually; its sides are very sharply marked. The disc shows a broad, shallow, physiological cupping, against the white ground of which the dark clump shows out most vividly. As compared with the little vein that passes under it coming from the nasal side, it requires 2 Ds. additional to focus upon its surface.

Fundus normal in all other respects.

———— —(Plate V, Fig. 3).

(49) Julia H.——. Aet. 19. Patient came for marginal phlyctenular keratitis. V was not up to normal on account of faint corneal opacities from previous phlyctenular trouble.

The ophthalmoscope showed clearly the center of the disc and the exit of the vessels covered by a clump of tissue. It was flame-like or flower-shaped, and showed a play of white and bluish-gray tints in its striations. At its center, over the deeper point of exit of the vessels, was an oval, rounded, more prominent clump of darker tissue. It resembled a hemp seed, or was like a rounded bunch of stamens to the flower-like membrane.

Fundus was entirely normal.

———— —(Plate V, Fig. 4).

(50) Miss Aggie B——. Aet. 15. Patient had asthenopia, corrected by + 1.25 D. $V = \frac{20}{28}$.

In her left eye the disc presented a dense, prominent, bluish-gray ridge of tissue covering the exit of the vessels. The artery and vein emerge from its upper edge. Two small arteries appear abruptly from behind its sharp inner border. Behind its outer border can be seen the main vein, which then penetrates the ridge to emerge below near the edge of the disc. The lower artery springs from its anterior face below. Very distinct parallax is had between the ridge and vein behind. The difference in focus amounts to 5 or 6 Ds., so that in the center the ridge projects quite well forward. Fundus normal. Her other eye had a delicate, semi-transparent film. (See case 17.)

———— —(Plate IX, Fig. 1).

(51) Bertha B——. Aet. 16. Came complaining of asthenopia.

With the proper glasses V was brought up to normal. The ophthalmoscope showed in the left eye a congenital underlying conus down and outward. What is rather rare in these cases, V was, however, brought up to $\frac{20}{28}$ with the correcting glasses. The center of the disc showed a glistening white clump of tissue which hid the point of exit of the vessels. From this there projected forward a rounded, conical stump, the atrophied remnant of the artery. Although difficult to focus upon its point, some 3 or 4 Ds. were required, indicating that it was about 1 mm. in length. It is an example which must correspond very closely to a microscopic slide I have from an ox's eye, where the atrophied remnant of a vessel projects about $1\frac{1}{2}$ mm. from the center of the optic disc.

DE SCHWEINITZ AND RANDALL—(Plate VIII, Fig. 1).

(52) Thos. H——. Aet. 22. Treated for severe serous iritis in the left eye. Cornea hazy; punctate descemititis; iris dull; fundus obscured, but nerve shows greenish and cupped, above it a reddish patch, probably a hemorrhage, and at its lower-inner side a large indistinct whitish area. $V = \frac{20}{100}$, while $R-V = \frac{20}{28}$. Anti-specific treatment and atropine.

One month later he was fitted with weak + glasses, and V became $\frac{14}{28}$ in this left eye. R normal. Ophthalmoscope showed the picture described below, and which was found unchanged at an examination made three years later, when the sketch was drawn.

The disc is cupped, showing somewhat greenish to its lower nasal side. A narrow conus to its lower temporal side, distinctly bounded by a pigment line. Above the disc considerable choroidal change and pigment deposit (this appearance is undoubtedly pathological). Tangent to the lower nasal margin of the disc is a regular, round, whitish area, whose diameter is about 1½ that of the disc. It is sharply bounded with abrupt and overhanging margins below and to the nasal side; toward the disc it shelves gradually and is peculiarly marked by mottled brown pigment. This area is greenish white and opalescent; it is depressed, requiring —3.0 D. to focus clearly; and is crossed horizontally by a large vein, which bends very sharply around the nasal border. Two very small and tortuous veins join this one at the middle of the patch. There seems little doubt of this being a small choroidal coloboma, although its position is unique.

A falciform outgrowth, semi-transparent and pale greenish or glistening white in tint, arises from the emergence of the vessels upon the disc, and extends its sharp edge some 3 D. forward into the vitreous. It curves up and inward more than 2 disc-diameters in length, and downward less than a disc-diameter. It loses itself at its extremities in fine threads stretching forward into the vitreous; the upper and longer extension being much the more marked and prominent. The membrane is thin, stretched, and non-vascular.

A small semi-detached vesicle, 3–4 D. in advance of the fundus, floats over the nasal margin of the disc (not shown in the sketch).

The retina has a marked striation at the posterior pole and glittering outlines along some of the vessels. The remainder of the fundus is normal and seen best with + 1.0 D. At this last examination V was $\frac{20}{8}$ with a weak + glass. The region of the coloboma had quantitative perception of light.

RANDALL—(Plate X, Fig. 3).

(53) Annie L——. Aet. 22. Came on account of dim sight in the right eye; left eye nearly normal. Thought this poor vision dated only back 2½ years, when sudden diplopia came on in the harvest field, from prostration by the heat—but without pain, headache or any illness (?). Girl stupid, and apparently hysterical. The ophthalmoscope revealed a flame-like membrane which covered nearly the lower half of the disc and spread downward-outward upon the retina, about one disc-diameter in width and two disc-diameters in length. It was glistening white, with a streaked reflex here and there in pale bluish-gray. It obscured the few vessels lying beneath it.

From its lower edge then continued still futher downward a rounded, elongated club-shaped projection. This appeared also to be adherent to the retinal surface (?) Its color was a pale greenish or bluish tint. Around its extremity were evidences of choroidal changes. Below the disc, about two disc-diameters, was a triangular patch of choroidal change.

The refraction (by ophth.) of the fundus was + 2.0 D.; of the thickest point of the membrane upon the disc + 4.0 D., and of the end of the club-like process + 8 0 D.

Fixation was poor; generally divergence.

GUENE—

(54) Soldier. Aet. 22. Presented the condition of micro-cornea, with convergent strabismus and rotatory nystagmus. The right eye revealed a very large, white disc, normal in contour above, below, and to the inner side; but with

a semi-circular expansion to the outer side (whether a myopic crescent or a sort of coloboma is not stated). The vessels, however, emerged at the line joining these two. To the outer side of the macula region was a large atrophic placque in the choroid.

The left eye, however, presented the condition of interest in our present study. The position of the papilla was occupied by a white patch slightly elongated in the horizontal diameter, and about the usual size of the disc. Its outer side is extended into a prolongation somewhat like a ribbon, stretching out about two and a half times the disc-diameter. This thins little by little, and is gradually lost in the retina. This prolongation and the patch itself, are distinctly striated. The vessels first appear not from the region of the disc, but from behind the upper edge of this band about half a disc-diameter away. The main artery curves around to the region of the disc and there divides into two branches, to be further distributed to the retina. In the region of the macula was a large atrophic placque as in the other eye. This description makes the case one very analagous to that of Dimmer's (No. 55), illustrated on Plate VI, Fig. 1.

DIMMER—(Plate VI, Figs. 1 and 2).

Patient was a young Jewish theological student, 24 years old. He was of frail physique, and vision had always been poor. Some months previous, vision in the right eye had began to fail still further, so that he was soon unable to read. He then noticed that the left eye had very poor vision also. The ophthalmoscope showed a very unusual example of congenital anomaly in each eye.

(55) LEFT EYE—(Plate VI, Fig. 1).

Only the inner half of the disc is seen. The outer half is covered by a prominent, whitish-gray mass of a quadrangular shape. This extends also about one disc-diameter over upon the adjacent retina. Its most prominent point lies over the lower-outer border of the disc, and requires + 3.5 D. to focus upon it. It is whitish-gray with a bluish tinge; has an asbestos luster; an irregular margin and uneven surface, and seems to be composed of numerous fibers interwoven together.

From its anterior surface there projects forward and downward a triangular process ending in a fine point (+ 8.0 D.). From all four corners and sides radiate forward numerous fine gray striæ (these require + 8 and + 9 Ds., but are not shown in the plate). These striæ inclose a funnel-shaped portion of the vitreous, with the wide mouth looking forward. (Profile in Plate 12, Fig. 4.)

From all four corners of the base of this mass, connective tissue bands spread out onto the retina. The three passing down, down and inward, up and inward are narrow, and border blood-vessels. That passing outward is broad and scythe-shaped, with its concave edge downward. This edge projects into the vitreous, so that in rolling the eye up one can see beneath it. Its upper edge slopes gradually into the general retinal level. This process is of about the same tint and texture as the quadrangular mass.

A short distance below this lower concave edge begins a narrow, club-shaped or tongue-shaped area about two disc-diameters in length, running downward. Its outer and upper edges are sharply defined and deeply pigmented. Its inner edge fades into the connective tissue band on this side. From this inner part an artery and vein arise. They curve across its upper half and then pass downward and outward to be distributed to the retina. This area has a yellowish-white surface, and is probably a rudimentary coloboma of the choroid. It corresponds to a sector-like defect found in the visual field above.

Five little circular rings of pigment inclosing white spots with a minute black dot at the center are observed. One is at the lower-inner disc border, one above the band passing outward, and three near the extremity of this band. Their explanation is not clear.

The lower and inner parts of the fundus are spotted with little groups of fine pigment dots.

V = counting fingers at 6 ft.

(56) RIGHT EYE—(Plate VI, Fig. 2).

Ophthalmoscope showed several fine opacities in the posterior cortex of the lens; near the inner periphery a web-like, triangular, grayish membrane directly behind the lens, and some fine punctate and some coarse flake-like floating opacities in the vitreous.

The disc could not be made out. Its site was covered by a bright, bluish-white, conical mass projecting diagonally forward and inward. Its fibrous texture and bluish tinge are similar to the mass in the other eye. The vessels all ramify from under the base of this cone. Connective tissue expansions pass from it, as in the other eye. A few narrow bands pass together downward and outward; and two broad, dense bands pass together directly outward. Around the base of the cone to the inner side the retina is detached. It is grayish-red, but not tremulous.

The most prominent part of the cone requires + 8.0 D. to focus (the general myopia of the fundus is about 2 D.)

From the upper edge of the cone a fine, clear, grayish fiber passes into the vitreous, forward and upward and outward. At its end is a small spindle-shaped swelling, requiring + 10 D. to focus. (This rudiment is omitted from the plate.)

Three of the curious spots, white with a black dot and ring, are seen—one below the cone, one directly outward, and one at the extremity of the lower connective tissue bands. Near the outer equator are some white reflecting spots; and scattered about the fundus are a few small groups of pigment.

V = counting fingers at 3 ft.

EWETZKI—

(57) Girl. Aet. 11. Left eye normal. The right eye was emmetropic, with V = $\frac{x}{xy}$. The lower segment of the visual field showed a triangular scotoma. The ophthalmoscope revealed in the fundus an oval mass of a whitish or bluish tint. Its rounded lower border covered the upper part of the disc. It extended upward and somewhat inward, dividing into three branches, which were slightly divergent. Its length was about two and a half disc-diameters, its width about that of the disc. The vessels were normal except that the superior ones were hid by the mass. The mass was immobile. Its general elevation required 5 D. to focus upon it clearly; its center was still more prominent, requiring 8 D.; and from this point it sent a thick process forward into the vitreous, which required over 10 D. to focus at all clearly upon it.

This case presents a striking similarity to those of Hersing (65) illustrated in Plate 7, Fig. 2; and Debierre (67), shown in profile on Plate 12, Fig. 9.

It is of especial interest as, lacking the characteristic remnant of the vessel itself, it joins these cases to the less typical forms like those of Dimmer.

BECKER (a)—

(58) Patient was a boy, from Professor Hebra's Clinic, utilized in the ophthalmoscopic class as a subject with normal fundus. V was normal. The ophthalmoscope showed the disc to be almost entirely covered by a grayish mass shaped like a star, or like a hand with outspread fingers. The disc contour could be made out only at places, and the vessels sprang abruptly from the edges of this mass, their central point being entirely hid.

The boy had never had any eye trouble.

——— —(a)

(59) Patient presented a picture somewhat similar to the above; but still more characteristic and unmistakable. The disc was covered by a bell-shaped, ribbed, grayish mass, much like the previous case, but more prominent. In addition, however, from the apex of this there projected forward a long cylindrical stalk, which reached to the neighborhood of the posterior surface of the lens. No distinct vessel could be detected in this strand. (Taken together this much resembled some little tree, the spreading roots of which were partially uncovered with earth and exposed). At the anterior extremity this widened into a goblet-like expansion, with some well-marked ribs, and delicate, membranous-like wall between them.

(Reuss also mentions having seen this case.)

REUSS—(Plate VII, Fig. 1).

(60) Lazar G——. Aet. 28. Patient was practically blind in his left eye, counting fingers at only a few inches, and only to the temporal side. The ophthalmoscope showed the fundus dotted with pigment spots around its periphery and reaching in to the disc at its nasal border. The spots were small, round, polygonal or spindle-shaped, only a few being stellate. There was no hemeralopia or concentric visual-field contraction, as in retinitis pigmentosa. The disc presents a marked picture (well given, I believe, in the plate). It is elliptical from above downward, and over twice the ordinary size. Its upper half is of the usual tint, its refraction + .50, and it is bounded below by a transverse curved border whose concavity looks downward. The lower half is deeply and sharply excavated, its refraction — 5.00, and its tint a glistening bluish white, without presenting the bright blue mottling usually seen in a deep physiological cupping. The vessels disappear abruptly at its edge, only three branches being visible upon its floor. A well-marked white scleral ring bounds it below and within. To the outer side is a well-marked pigment ring. We have, in other words, a fairly characteristic example of coloboma of the optic nerve sheath.

From the curved border line dividing (or bounding?) the disc, and to its inner side, there springs forward a thick, conical, stalagmite-shaped body, of a bluish-white tint. Its base resting upon the sloping edge, it resembles a little tower built on the very brink of a precipitous crag. It requires an additional + 5.00 D to focus upon its rounded end. From this end there pass forward an innumerable number of the finest striae, slightly diverging. They have an appearance like fine foldings or striations in a membrane, and the general effect is as if one were looking down into the spreading mouth of a funnel. This is no doubt the visible wall of the central canal.

Within this and from the end of the conical process there pass forward two
fine filaments, evidently obliterated vessels, having a wavy course, diverging
slightly, and being lost in the vitreous. The retinal vessels coming from
the disc proper all emerge from under the base of this conical process.

Upon the posterior surface of the lens, in its upper outer quadrant, are three
opacities, lying outside the capsule. Two round spots are peripheral, and
joining these is a triangular patch passing inward, its apex reaching to the
posterior pole. This spot appears to have considerable thickness, and to
project into the vitreous, but no strand passes backward from it to connect
with the deeper remains. The right eye presents the peripheral pigment
spots, a grayish-red disc, and thin vessels. He reads J. No. 17 at 3 in.
slowly and with difficulty. Visual field normal.

(61) Adolph R——. Aet. 15. Boy had never seen well, right eye being the
poorer.

$V = \frac{8}{80}$, Hm. 3.00 D. $V = \frac{8}{30}$.   The fundus presented a general choroiditis, being spotted with round pigment groups, especially abundant toward
the periphery. Most of these are paler in the center; but no atrophic
patches are present. Some stellate and irregular patches were also found.
The macula region is nearly intact.

From one of the primary arterial branches upon the disc springs a translucent, grayish strand of moderate thickness, which passes directly forward.
This rapidly thins out (spindle-shaped) into a fine fiber, whose end is lost in
a small cloud-like opacity occupying the more forward part of the central
canal of the vitreous, slightly inward and below the posterior pole of the
lens.

Lying upon the edge of the disc are five rounded, bluish-white clumps,
the two larger being the size of about $\frac{1}{4}$ of the area of the disc. They are
somewhat translucent, appear to be formed of most minute nodules or
shreds, and resemble a ball of loosely packed snow whose edges are melt-
ing. They require 1 D. additional to focus clearly, and give a parallactic
movement with the vessels passing beneath them.

(This is the same patient whose left eye is described as case 157.)

BAYER (b)—

(62) Man. Aet 31. The ophthalmoscope revealed a bell-shaped, transparent
mass, which rested upon the optic papilla. Its anterior, narrowed portion
projected forward into the clear vitreous. From the edges of this bell-
shaped mass streamed out numerous fine, thread-like filaments.

The author thinks possibly that there had been here a fluid distension of
the canal, and rupture. He explains the basal portion remaining and the
fine threads floating forward, in this way.

(63) Patient was a girl. Aet. 14. $V = \frac{1}{2}$; no contraction of the visual field.
The ophthalmoscope revealed a white plate or membrane covering the optic
disc. Its edges were marked with pigment deposits, and from its lower
border emerged the central vessels of the retina. The picture presented
reminded one very greatly of the cases of coloboma of the optic nerve
sheath. Projecting forward from this plate upon the disc was a conical,
thin-walled, translucent mass somewhat similar to that observed in the pre-

vious case. It also presented numerous fine, thread-like filaments passing forward and downward. Below the disc, and further forward on the floor of the globe, was an irregular, tent-shaped elevation, formed by a delicate membrane of a bluish-white tint, and crossed by several small vessels. To this membrane were attached many of the filaments which sprang from the mass upon the disc site. That this was not a detachment of the retina was quite evident. It was probably a remnant of the early mesoderm process that comes in here.

The retinal vessels presented quite an unusual arrangement in their division and distribution.

BRAILEY—

(64) Florence R——. Aet. 3¼. Child delicate and sickly. R. eye had been congested and painful. Ordinary tests proved it to be blind. On admission the anterior chamber was found to be shallow; the pupil irregular from several posterior synchiæ, but the lens clear. It had the appearance of a case of detached retina, and being somewhat painful was enucleated by Mr. Hutchinson. On equatorial section the posterior lens capsule was seen to be covered by a bluish-white fibrous opacity. This opacity spread out laterally as far as the ora serrata retinæ. It was deficient but at one point, through which the clear lens could be seen.

From its center a slender, flattened white cord springs, to pass back to the region of the disc. Posteriorly it joins the apex of a quadrangular pyramid which completely hides the disc, and which seems to be formed of detached retina. The sides of this mass are grooved in the direction of its long axis, and its base slopes off into the general retinal level. In the groove between its upper and outer angles, at its base, is seen a darker colored minute patch, apparently the yellow spot.

Histologically, cornea, sclera, ciliary body and lens are normal. The ciliary processes are overlaid by an indistinct, finely fibrillated tissue in which are numerous easily stained corpuscles with dot-like nuclei, intermixed with a few prolongations of pigment cells from beneath. The columnar cells of the pars ciliaris, with their elongated nuclei, are lengthened so as to make the layer thicker than usual.

HERSING —(Plate VII, Fig. 2).

(65) Girl 11 years old. Came on account of strabismus convergens concomitans of right eye. V = counting fingers at about 1 ft., with excentric fixation. L. eye Hm. .75 D. V = ⅚.

R. eye—ophthalmoscope showed the lens transparent, but its posterior capsule presented clearly numerous radiating striations. In the center at the posterior pole was a white mass the size of a pin-head. From this there passed backward a thick, freely moving strand, which appeared either grayish-white or pinkish, according to the incidence of the light. Near its posterior end it swelled out to the size of a pea, then narrowed again, and then immediately broadened to spread out into a tripod resting upon the disc. This covered the outer half or more of the papilla. One prominent, thick and rounded process, about one disc-diameter in length, passed directly upward; one narrowed process, about 2 disc-diameters in length, passed downward and inward; the third process, narrow and 3 to 4 disc-diameters in length, passed downward and outward. The ends of these two faded gradually into the retina. The processes were grayish-blue in tint. The retina is lifted to every-where pass over these folds. Some of the vessels emerge from the free portion of the disc, but their upper branches curve over the rounded upper process. Other vessels spring from beneath the folds, and course upon and over them. This is most clearly shown on the long temporal edge, and upon the inner edges where the two lower processes meet.

The choroid presents a few small groups of pigment, especially below, between the two lower processes. The vitreous is clear, but fluidified.

The entire picture resembles an upright stand, with its tripod base resting on the disc, and the shaft supporting the lens.

EVERSBUSCH (a)—

(66) Boy of 14 years. His left eye was practically normal, but the right eye was highly amblyopic.

The ophthalmoscope revealed at the posterior pole a bluish clump the size of a pin-head. From this radiated some 15–20 fine processes upon the posterior capsule, while a larger undulating strand passed directly backward. This soon enlarged to a club-shaped mass, which, in the middle of the vitreous, broadened out into a funnel-shaped, bluish-gray membrane. The base of this covered the lower half of the disc, and the retina below.

At some places it passed abruptly, and at other places gradually into the general retinal level. The upper half of the disc was normal, and the vessels springing from it were regularly distributed to the upper (normal) portions of the fundus. The membrane formed a sort of a triangular tent-like fold directly downward; and from a cleft in this, arterial and venous vessels emerged to be distributed to the retina below. Near the base of the lower fold were pigment patches, and disturbances in the choroid. The vitreous was clear. The resemblance to Hersing's case is striking.

DEBIERRE—(Plate XII, Fig. 9).

(67) Girl of 7 years. Child had strab. conv. of right eye. V = counting fingers at 3 meters with excentric fixation. H of about ¾ D. by the ophthalmoscope.

By oblique illumination there presented a slight central haze of the cornea. Five well marked fibers of a persistent pupillary membrane sprang from the face of the iris to be inserted into a cresent shaped, dotted, dark band of opacity upon the anterior face of the crystalline lens. Upon the posterior face was found a white triangular placque, occupying the lower inner sector, covering about ⅓ of the posterior capsule. The ophthalmoscope showed a pyramidal, whitish or grayish mass, covering the disc. Its triangular base was obliquely directed, its longest axis being from below at the nasal side, to the temporal side above.

It resembles the case of Hersing (65) very closely. From this pyramid, a narrowed, rounded, dark cord, passes forward in a drooping curve through the vitreous. When near the lens it spreads out into a fan-shaped, or funnel-shaped expansion to be inserted upon the whitish plate upon the posterior capsule.

The cord floats with sinuous movements upon movement of the eyeball.

BERGER (A. M.)—

(68) Woman. Aet. 60. In the left eye was found a narrow canal reaching to the posterior pole of the lens and terminating there in an enlarged or expanded

end. This enlarged part has a greenish gray tint. The middle portion is movable and spirally curved. It is fixed at the disc by an enlargement in form of a funnel, which covers the lateral portion of the papilla, and terminates in a fine point directed toward the physiological cup. Resembles the cases of Hersing and Debierre to a great extent.

SAEMISCH (b)—

(69) Girl of 20 years. Came on account of a slight injury to the right eye. In the left eye the ophthalmoscope showed the lower two-thirds of the disc free and of a normal appearance. The upper third of the disc and the retina above, was covered by the base of a tubular body which projected forward into the vitreous. This base formed a elongated oval, its long diameter placed vertically and about 2 disc-diameters in length. It was formed of a delicate, bluish-white membrance, which passed gradually into the neighboring retina, in a way resembling a small tent. This pale bluish membrane had some branches of the retinal vessels passing over it; while other branches of the superior vessels passed under it to again appear at its opposite border, and spread out over the normal retina. The remainder of the fundus was normal. From this oval base an oval body of the same size was continued forward for a short distance; this then rapidly narrowed to a cylindrical shaft of about one-third the diameter of the basal portion, this passed directly forward about three-fourths of the distance to the lens, and there terminated in an enlarged, rounded, knob like extremity. This narrowed anterior portion carried no blood vessels. The entire body showed no distinct undulations on movements of the eye V was normal, and patient had never had any eye trouble.

GROUP E—REMNANT ATTACHED TO THE DISC.

This group forms the first subdivision of the large class of the ordinary forms of persistent hyaloid artery, where a narrow strand passes through the vitreous.

The group is the largest of all these that we have arranged for purposes of convenience. It is characterized by a strand arising from the disc, passing forward for a greater or less distance, and terminating by an end which floats free in the vitreous. Usually the origin of the strand can be traced clearly to the central artery, although some take origin from a branch upon the disc, and in Mooren's case from a branch *outside* the disc. Occasionally its origin can not be sharply traced to the artery, but its movements show it to be fixed at the end upon or near the disc.

The length is of course variable; they may subdivide into two or three branches, and may terminate either in knob-like swellings, in fine fibrillæ, or in delicate tapering points.

Their color varies from grayish, bluish, brownish to black—to some extent modified by the method of illumination.

With a very strict classification, some of the cases in the previous group would be classed here ; for example the cases of Dimmer, Reuss, Becker, Bayer, and Saemisch. But in these cases the clumps of tissue upon and about the disc are of greater interest than the strands passing forward into the vitreous.

I am strongly of the opinion that a delicate remnant of this sort is a very common occurrence in the human eye. I refer to the instances where an extremely delicate, short strand projects from the disc. It is usually white or faintly bluish in tint, and ends in a fine point, or delicate knob. I figure four on Plate IX. Since that plate was drawn I have seen two others, quite symmetrical, in the two eyes of a young woman. They closely resembled the Fig. 3 on Plate IX, being, however, shorter and somewhat thicker. This makes six in all that I have seen of this delicate variety, indicating that they must be common. In fact I believe that they must be frequently overlooked. So delicate are they that they are perfectly invisible by the indirect method, (even when one knows the remain to be there), and may even be overlooked by a careless, routine, direct examination. The necessities of graphic representation compel me to bring them out much more clearly in the plate than they really appear.

All the cases seen have been in normal eyes, or at most in those with only refractive errors.

I shall not be surprised, after this is published, to hear that many observers, with whom the direct method is a favorite, have seen numerous similar cases, but have not thought them worthy of publication.

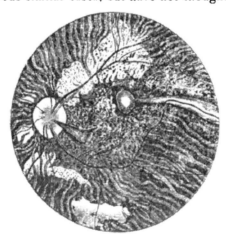

This cut, taken from Stellwag's large work on Diseases of the Eye, is a very good representation of the short remnants ending in broadened, frayed-out extremities, floating free in the vitreous. This cut is no doubt a picture of Reuss's case (105), as well as Stellwag's (106), for it is almost certain that these two cases are really the same, reported independently by these two observers; both being in the same city—Vienna.

FIG. 2 (STELLWAG).

MEISSNER—

(70) This was the first recorded example of this anomaly observed in the *human* subject, and was seen post-mortem.

Cadaver of an old man. On dissecting the eye there was found a tolerably thick, white process, about 1 line in length, emerging from the center of the disc, and projecting directly forward into the vitreous.

ULRICH—

(71) Girl of 7 years. She had typical retinitis pigmentosa in both eyes, hemeralopia, and the parents were related.

Left eye showed a conical, translucent process projecting from the physiological cup, and extending a short distance into the vitreous.

(72) Right eye showed a distinct, translucent strand projecting from the physiological cup. It had not the well-marked conical appearance presented in the other eye.

HIRSCHBERG (b)—

(73) H. B——. Adult. Left eye showed with the ophthalmoscope a M. of 1 D. This also revealed a rudimentary hyaloid. From over the upper branch of the central artery, which divides very near the middle of the disc, there projects a short, delicate, club-shaped process. This rapidly dwindles in the vitreous, to a fine terminal point.

OETTINGEN (a)—

(74 and 75) Patient an adult. Similar condition in *both* eyes.

There emerged from the main trunk of the central vessels upon the disc a short, grayish-white strand. This broadened to a membranous expansion 1-2 ‴ in width, which reached forward to the center of the vitreous. This expansion partially hid the disc, although careful focussing showed that it did not lie in the same level.

————— —(b)

(76 and 77) Patient a young girl.

The ophthalmoscope showed a gray, conical-shaped process, springing from the trunk of the central artery upon the disc. The process is thicker than the artery, and projects but a short distance into the vitreous.

The condition was exactly similar in both eyes.

————— —(b)

(78) Patient a recruit. Aet. 25. Left eye had poor V. The ophthalmoscope revealed a dark strand springing from the branch of the central artery upon the lower-inner part of the optic disc. There was a small central physiological cup.

The strand passes forward in a straight line through the center of the vitreous. Its caliber remains about that of the main branch of the vein. It showed single contoured. It terminates with a button-like extremity, being free, about 1-2 mm. behind the posterior surface of the lens. This terminal enlargement was about the size of a large pin-head.

The strand appeared black and opaque in its entire course, except its posterior portion, which showed translucent and grayish-white by accurate focussing.

The strand did not move about in a fluidified vitreous, its apparent movement being due to the parallax between the different parts.

Patient had never any entoptic phenomena.

COWELL—

(79) Sarah A. B——. Aet. 32. Presented herself on account of a previous attack of iritis, which had left two or three posterior synechiæ. On ophthal-

moscopic examination of the left eye the optic disc was perfectly healthy. From its center, at the point of emergence and bifurcation of the arteria centralis, of which it seemed to be a continuation, there projected forward an opaque filament of a grayish color. It tapered to a point, and was apparently about 2½ lines in length.

LITTLE—

(80) Miss W——. (Sister of case 134). Patient is myopic. The ophthalmoscope showed in the left eye a slight remnant of the hyaloid artery at the disc.

DeBeck—(Plate IX, Fig. 2).

(81) Ennis B——. Aet. 11 (colored). Child came with phlyctenular keratitis (marginal). $V = \frac{28}{8}$.

Ophthalmoscope showed a broad and deep physiological cupping, characteristically mottled.

From the main trunk of the central artery on the floor of this excavation there sprang forward a thin, faintly grayish strand. It passed but a short distance forward, was extremely narrow, but rounded, and ended in a tapering point. It resembled more than any thing else a fine quill toothpick. No movement in it could be detected, but as it was very short and difficult to keep in view, this may have been overlooked.

——— —(Plate IX, Fig. 4).

(82) Man. Aet. about 25. This case was seen in Dr. Dimmer's ophthalmoscopic class in Vienna in the spring of 1883. The man had been brought in from another clinic to present to the beginners a normal fundus, and this anomaly in his *right* eye was only thus accidentally discovered. Dr. Randall of Philadelphia, who was a fellow student at the time, may remember the case when he sees the sketch. Here a whitish clump hid the exit of the vessels, and from it there projected forward a pale, bluish, rounded strand, the atrophied artery. It had a wavy, sinuous movement, the vitreous just in front of the disc being fluid. It was probably 2 or 3 mm. at least in length. V seemed to be normal, as the man claimed.

——— —(Plate IX, Fig. 3).

(83) Ammie B——. Aet. 28. Patient came for refractive trouble. With + .75 s. $\supset + 1.00$ c. 90°, $V = \frac{28}{8}$.

Fundus and disc were normal in the left eye; but from the exact point of division of the central artery into its primary branches, there sprang a pale, bluish gray, rounded strand, about the diameter of one of the blood vessels of fourth magnitude. It passed forward and downward, and terminated with a rounded, slightly knobbed extremity. It oscillated gently on movements of the eyeball.

REMAK—(Plate V, Fig. 6).

(84). Middle-aged man. Came on account of beginning presbyopia. Both eyes were emmetropic and vision normal. In the right eye the ophthalmoscope showed a transversly ovoid disc, with a conus downward ⅓ the width of the disc diameter. The vessels emerged from the disc irregularly and widely separated. Those passing downward were hid by a delicate, dark gray membrane. This passed forward and downward and gradually narrowed to a fine point, seen best with $+ 5.0$ D.

With $+ 8.0$ D. a free body could be seen in the vitreous. This resembled four little drops hanging together, or a couple of delicate dumb-bells crossing by the handles.

DeBeck—(Plate IX, Figs. 5 and 6).

Miss Mary M——. Aet. 22. Patient came on account of poor vision. R. eye $V = \frac{20}{200}$. Myopia of 3 or 4 Ds. not improved materially by glasses. L. eye $V =$ only to counting fingers at 10 to 12 feet. Myopia of same degree as in R. eye.

(85) RIGHT EYE (fig. 5), showed an average disc; to its outer side was a narrow crescent of beginning atrophy, to the inner side were several annular groups of pigment spots (but one shown in the figure), and from the center of the disc sprang a hyaloid remnant. It began at the point of exit of the vessels, which it veiled, as a soft, thin, nearly transparent grayish membrane. It passed forward, becoming thicker, but remaining flattened, and terminated in a somewhat broader frayed end, which showed perfectly black against the red background. It oscillated very freely on movements of the eye, and focussing upon its vibrating end was extremely difficult, but certainly 8 to 10 Ds. were necessary to bring it into sharp view.

(86) LEFT EYE (fig. 6).—The disc resembled the other eye, with a similar narrow atrophic crescent. To the inner side were two small patches of choroidal atrophy. Along the border of the disc nearest to these was a short, thick band of pigment. At the macula was a central coloboma (?) perfectly circular, and about twice the diameter of the disc. The point of exit of the vessels upon the disc was completely covered by a funnel-shaped, pale, gray expansion. This passed forward, gradually tapering, became cylindrical, a trifle thicker than the largest vein, and terminated in a very distinct round knob, nearly twice the diameter of the shaft. It moved slowly to and fro on movements of the eye, and 12 Ds. would focus clearly upon its point.

Lens and vitreous in both eyes were clear.

Berger (A. M.)—

(87) Man. Aet. 45. Patient had myopia of ¼.

The ophthalmoscope showed a dark strand springing from the temporal side of the disc. It passed with a slight sinuous course forward into the vitreous, having a length about equal to one disc-diameter. It terminated with a somewhat frayed-out free end, which moved widely on movements of the eye.

Ewers—

(88–89) Patient presented a similar appearance in each eye. A bluish-gray strand was found running backward through the center of the vitreous, in the axis of the eye. It was not connected with the lens, its anterior extremity being freely movable. It gradually tapered to a fine filament as it approached the disc, becoming invisible and its direct connection with the disc itself could not be made out. It must have been attached somewhere here, however, for this formed a fixed point during the undulations of the strand.

Callan—

Examined some five hundred colored children in two public schools in New York city. He found among these two cases of anomalous retinal vessels projecting into the vitreous, and one case of remains of the hyaloid artery.

(90) Thos. M. K——. Aet. 18 (colored). Patient myopic (— 30 in.) each eye. The R. eye has media and fundus normal, and V = $\frac{20}{30}$, with the correcting concave 30. Left eye examined with the ophthalmoscope showed a slightly turbid vitreous. Arising from the lower main arterial trunk, on the optic disc near the choroidal ring, was a small thread-like vessel. It extended forward to very near the posterior capsule of the lens. It presented a dark contour, but was evidently destitute of blood. It moved freely and widely with any movement of the eyeball.

V was only $\frac{12}{30}$ (with the correcting concave 30), owing to the slight turbidity of the fluidified vitreous.

MOOREN (a)—

(91) Patient was a peasant in middle life. The left eye presented extreme strabismus divergens; the iris was tremulous from fluidity of the vitreous, and V was poor. He read T. No. 20 only partly and with difficulty, and glasses did not improve. The disc and retinal vessels were rather rudimentary. To the *outer side* of the disc, there sprang from one of the arterial *branches* a small, grayish-blue strand, which passed forward through the vitreous. The filament was straight, only along its upper surface having slight wave-like curves, and reached nearly to the posterior surface of the lens.

It moved slowly about on any rapid movement of the eye.

——— (b)—

(92) Another case was observed in which the appearances were very similar to the above. Instead, however, of the strand having the very unusual point of insertion as recorded above, it here sprang from the main branch of the central artery upon the disc.

PERRIN—(Plate X, Fig. 1).

(93) The author gives in his atlas a colored figure, which we copy. The eye had H. of 4.00 Ds. V = only $\frac{1}{200}$.

At the posterior pole of the lens was a small, brilliant point, indicating the site of the previous attachment of the artery. The ophthalmoscope showed a large, white disc. From the center of this sprang a straight, smooth, cylindrical strand, passing directly forward through the vitreous toward the lens. This terminated in a rounded, knob-like end, about three times the diameter of the trunk. The trunk was bluish-gray. The rounded extremity a bluish-white.

In concentric bands about the disc were evidences of choroidal disturbances, and streaks of pigment.

CARRERAS–ARAGO—(Plate X, Fig. 2).

(94) Mrs. Rosa B——. Aet. 51. Came on account of failing vision, with annoying shadows in the left eye. V = $\frac{3}{100}$.

The ophthalmoscope showed some faint striæ at the posterior pole of the lens. The disc was a very dark pink, with an unusually wide and deep physiological cup. The vessels sprang from the edges of this, and presented nothing unusual, except four filiform arteries which emerged from the same point as the hyaloid rudiment, and passed together downward and outward.

From the lower-outer edge of the cup sprang a round thin strand. This passed forward, gradually growing thicker until it was somewhat larger than the main veins, and then terminated in a rounded, club-shaped extremity, about three times the diameter of the trunk. It was milky white in color, and gave a glistening reflex. It made wide and almost incessant vermicular movements on the least move of the eyeball.

Fundus was normal.

PFLUEGER—

(95) Marie G——. Aet. 12. Patient has total irideremia, both eyes. (Mother has the same condition.) $V = \frac{1}{10}$. Reads moderate sized type.

The ophthalmoscope shows a sinuous strand running forward through the vitreous. It springs from just below the disc, with a slightly funnel-shaped base apparently connected with a retinal vein (?). It extends directly forward, becoming gradually narrower in its course through the center of the vitreous. Near the lens it again very slightly enlarges, and ends directly behind the lens, without being connected to the posterior pole. The strand is dark gray, and distinctly double-contoured. It is surrounded by a delicate, translucent, faint-gray sheath during its entire length. It shows very free and extensive movements on moving the eye; again resuming its central position when the eye comes to rest.

(96 and 97) Alexander G——. Aet. 5 mos. Brother of the above case (Marie G). This patient has also total irideremia—both eyes. Has in addition a small anterior polar cataract. The ophthalmoscope reveals in each eye a sinuous, waving, gray strand exactly analogous to the condition found in his elder sister's eyes.

SULZER—

(98) Young man of 17 years. R. eye had H. $V = \frac{5}{8}$, with + 1.5 D. The ophthalmoscopic appearances normal. L. eye has M. With — 5.0 D., $V = \frac{5}{8}$.

The ophthalmoscope showed an ovoid disc, with a dark, mottled pigment ring, and a narrow underlying conus. From the lower margin there emerged, with a sharp curve, a glistening white strand. This became of a dark gray color, and passed with a sinuous course forward and downward through the vitreous, and apparently ended free.

There were numerous other anomalies. A single fine shred of persistent pupillary membrane, adherent to a pigment speck on the anterior capsule, and to the smaller circle of the iris. There was a posterior cortical opacity at the periphery of the lower-inner quadrant. Behind the lens, back of this opacity, were two flat, striated, white bands, 2 to 2½ mm. wide, and about the length of the corneal diameter, coming up from the ciliary region and running toward the posterior pole. The one to the temporal side had a mother-of-pearl gleam, and carried a little blood vessel upon its anterior face. The one to the nasal side, seen through the lenticular opacity, appeared as a dull, gray strand, with irregular edges. Finally, on the floor of the vitreous was a tubular membrane beginning in front of the equator a little to the outer side, with a base about three times that of the disc. It passed back, and was inserted below the disc. It was funnel-shaped at each end, and about the diameter of the disc at its central portion, where its refraction was + 4.0 and + 5.0 D., showing that its surface was 3 mm. in front of the retina. It was steel gray, or the color of detached retina, and carried both arterial and venous branches. This was no doubt a remnant of the early mesoderm involution that formed the vitreous.

CARTER (b)—

(99) Mary L——. Aet. 30. Had asthenopia, with impaired vision in the left eye. With + 2.50 D., vision equal to one-third. With the mirror a floating body was detected, not seen in the inverted image. With the direct image a delicate film was detected, attached posteriorly to the disc, but its direct attachment to the vascular system not to be clearly made out. Passing forward it formed a delicate *double* cylinder, each tube of which terminated anteriorly in a little knob. These required + 8.00 D. to be clearly focussed.

Near the equator a large patch of choroidal atrophy was discovered. It was probably also congenital.

STREATFIELD—

(100) Emma S——, married. Aet. 48. Came on account of the inflamed, nearly blind left eye, which also squinted outward, and showed a ciliary staphyloma.

From the center of the disc there sprang a broad, opaque band, which passed forward through the center of the vitreous. Its anterior end narrowed to a fine point, which turned to one side, and was not inserted into the posterior lens capsule.

The author notes the possibility of this being a pathological product.

REUSS—

(101) Boleslav M——. Aet. 27. Came with retinitis of left eye. The right eye had been practically blind since earliest childhood. In this eye the ophthalmoscope showed a hyaloid remain. From the central artery there sprang a thin, transparent strand about the diameter of a secondary vein. It passed forward through the vitreous, with a slight curve like a loose rope, divided into two small branches near its extremity, and ended in the vicinity of the posterior surface of the lens. It oscillated gently on movements of the eyeball. The disc was blurred, veins slightly enlarged, but V was not improved on dismissal, with V = 1 in the other (left) eye.

LANG—

(102) Patient well-developed man of 21. R. eye has always had poor vision. He reads J. No. 16 poorly, and with — 7 D. V = $\frac{6}{60}$ ($\frac{20}{200}$).

The ophthalmoscope shows a large band of connective tissue starting from the center of the disc. It passes directly forward, and when about a quarter of the way through the vitreous it divides into three branches. The main or central branch passes forward to be attached to the posterior pole of the lens; the second comes forward directly above this nearly to the upper edge of the back of the lens; the third runs horizontally forward and inward, but does not reach much beyond the equator of the globe. They are all white by direct examination, but by oblique illumination, the one that follows the course of the hyaloid artery is brownish in color.

Around the disc is considerable choroidal atrophy, and white bands border most of the vessels. That portion of the disc not covered by the connective tissue bands is of a dark color. At the upper and inner part of the fundus is some choroidal pigmentation, with atrophy.

Reuss—

(103) Nehemias N——. Aet. 52. Patient was a Russian upon whom an iridectomy in the right eye had been performed on account of acute glaucoma, with clouding of the vitreous, and incipient cortical cataract. Ten months later he was examined, the acute symptoms having disappeared after the operation, and the tension now being normal. Examination difficult on account of the hazy lens, but revealed a deep glaucoma excavation. At the lower inner border, there sprang from one of the arterial branches, just before it disappeared over the edge, a double contoured, nearly transparent strand. Close to its source it gave off at an acute angle a small branch whose end could not be followed. The main branch passed directly forward through the center of the vitreous. It terminated in a small knob-like end not far from the posterior surface of the lens, but without making any attachment to the posterior pole.

(104) August Sp——. Aet. 52. The old man had several times been used as a subject in the ophthalmoscopic course, on account of a characteristic choroiditis, without his anomaly being noted. In his left eye there sprang from the artery in the center of the disc a grayish strand, not cylindrical but flattened transversely. It passed a short distance forward, and rapidly thinning seemed to end here in the vitreous. In reality it broke up into a number of excessively fine, pellucid fibrillæ, which were well made out by examination with sunlight. Three of these, slightly diverging, passed directly forward, another passed forward and inward. Their ending could not be made out on account of their extreme tenuity. The vitreous was filled with the finest of cloud-like opacities. Fundus had general choroiditis, with pigment groups, gray disc, and thin vessels. V only perception of light.

(105) August D——. Aet. 17. Boy in the alms house, used as material in the ophthalmoscope course. In the right eye there was present a well-marked posterior polar cataract. It was 5 rayed, the upper-inner one dividing into two branches, the others ending broad, rounded, and knob-like. It lay upon the posterior surface of the capsule. From the center of the papilla sprang a strand with a club-shaped, translucent base; it ran a short distance into the vitreous, becoming dark gray, and ended with a knob-like swelling. From this a larger number of minute fibers streamed forward like a little broom. Among these were five more distinct and thicker than the rest. No connection with the posterior polar cataract could be detected; in fact the strand seemed to be directed more toward a point to the temporal side of the lens center.

In the fundus, about three disc-diameters to the temporal side of the papilla, is a horizontal fold of bluish white tint. It begins with a rounded swelling; from this it passes thin and narrow; further out it broadens, and its peripheral termination is not visible. Retinal vessels pass over it. The choroid is atrophic; presents irregular whitish and yellowish patches; has a few pigment groups, some like those of retinitis pigmentosa; the disc is grayish-red, and the vessels thin.

Stellwag—

(106) S. undoubtedly figures the same case in his " Treatise on the Diseases of the

Eye," N. Y. Translation of 1873, p. 134, fig. 26. In this cut the nearly transparent base is not shown, but the anterior expanded end is well shown, corresponding very closely with Reuss's description. The curious remnant in the retina leaves no doubt that the case, an asylum inmate, is the same, independently described by these two observers, both of whom are in the same University—in Vienna. (See Fig. 2.)

Magnus—(Plate X, Fig. 4).

(107) Mathias K——. Aet. 49. Came on account of asthenopia. The left eye had $V = \frac{20}{40}$ with $+ 1.25$ D.; the right eye only counted fingers and had always seen poorly. The ophthalmoscope showed the media clear. The disc was distinctly egg-shaped, the point directed horizontally inward. It was surrounded by a very broad, mottled ring of pigment clumps. The pointed segment of the disc was covered with a white membrane, which almost completely hid the point of exit of all the vessels. This was the expanded base of a conical, bluish-white process which projected into the vitreous. It terminated in a quadrangular, bluish, club-like head, from which passed still further forward three narrow, fine dark strands. The two springing from the angles of this clump pass to the inner edge of the lens, but their insertion can not be made out. The third and finest can not be readily traced, and floats freely. A narrow white strand passes inward in the retina. It branches and curves slightly downward, and is apparently an obliterated retinal vessel.

Becker (a)—

(108) Patient presented a hyaloid remain arising from the center of the disc, which was otherwise free. The anterior extremity of this strand did not reach the lens, but broke up into a number of fine fibers, which terminated in a number of small white masses and membranes, occupying this part of the vitreous. The whole appearance was much like the head of a cauliflower.

(Reuss had also seen this case, and adds a few points to Prof. Becker's short notice.)

Kipp—

(109) F. C——. Aet. 60. Came with small splinter on conjunctiva. Complaining also of poor vision, an ophthalmoscopic examination was made. The choroid was slightly atrophied in both eyes. In the right eye there emerged from the center of the optic disc a vessel the size of a primary branch of the central artery. It at once twisted itself into a small loop, the details of which are neither described nor figured in the original. This loop was of a light red color. This was then continued as a straight dark cord, surrounded by a translucent envelope, which passed directly forward as far as the center of the vitreous. Its anterior end became about three times as broad as the trunk, and was somewhat flattened laterally. It here divided into three short branches, the free extremities of which were bulbous. The *loop* evidently contained blood, for pressure on the globe produced pulsation in it, as well as in the retinal arteries. In the left eye was present an anomalous retinal vessel, one of that not extremely rare variety which passes out into the vitreous, and then bends back to twine about itself and return to the fundus.

HARLES A. OLIVER, M.D.,
1507, LOCUST STREET,
PHILADELPHIA.

VANLAIR—

(110) Child. Aet. 4. The right eye was the seat of severe pain. On examination the fundus gave back a glistening, yellowish reflex. This was from a richly vascular tumor occupying the entire posterior portion of the eyeball. The eye was enucleated; 2½ months later the growth had returned, filling the entire orbit; and three months later the child died.

The microscopic examination showed the disc infiltrated by a soft tissue with alveolar arrangement. The posterior portion of the vitreous was filled by a soft, pulpy, clouded mass. Under the play of a fine stream of water this soft material was washed away, and left only an intricate net-work of blood-vessels having an attachment only at the disc. Through this mass passed the hyaloid artery to the anterior part of the vitreous, which was still normal. This vessel gave off numerous side branches. The author calls this a " granulome telangiectasique:" it was probably the ordinary glioma retinæ.

What makes this case of special interest is, that the author regards this growth as having its origin in this persistent hyaloid artery, with which it was so curiously connected. His view is, however, not conclusive. The possibility and even probability, that this vessel, which from its position and course so resembled the hyaloid artery, may have been a new formation, can not be excluded.

GROUP F—STRAND ATTACHED TO THE DISC, AND A VESTIGE ON THE LENS.

This forms a small group. It resembles the previous one in having a strand springing forward from the disc and ending free in the vitreous; differs in presenting in addition a distinct remnant at the posterior pole of the lens, indicating the former attachment of the artery at this point.

This attachment is not always central; it may sometimes be excentric. This figure, taken from Loring's Text-book of Ophthalmoscopy—and somewhat elaborated—is a very excellent illustration of this group. The profile view is the only one that gives a fair idea of these cases. Any sort of front view is very unsatisfactory, and sometimes really impracticable.

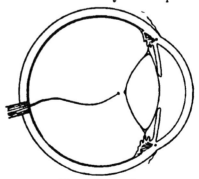

FIG. 3 (LORING).

This group is only of importance as illustrating that in the process of obliteration, the artery may divide at some point in its course through the vitreous; and that then the process of obliteration may stop before either end has entirely disappeared. It is also useful to more handily divide up the material.

The case of Unterharnscheidt (116), is of interest as showing the possibility of this rupture taking place years after birth. In this case resulting from the axial elongation in progressive myopia.

Some few cases in Groups D and E might properly be included here, but their predominant interest is there.

REMAK—(Plate V, Fig. 5).

(111) Miss V——. Aet. 22. Came on account of conjunctivitis. Right eye had always been amblyopic, and now presented marked divergent strabismus. With the ophthalmoscope the eye was myopic to an extreme degree. Left normal. Just up and inward from the posterior pole was inserted a very fine filament which passed back a short distance into the vitreous.

The disc was round, with a continuous and broad pigment ring, which sent out two pigment outliers, one in, the other directly outward. Directly downward was an elongated rectangular area, white, and bounded and crossed by pigment lines. This is probably a small coloboma of the choroid, of unusual shape. The point of exit of the vessels is covered by a small, round, grayish mass of tissue; and from this there passes forward a grayish, translucent strand. This begins with rather a broad base, tapers gradually, and ends as a fine fiber in the vitreous. It moves slowly on movements of the eyeball.

——— —(Plate VIII, Fig. 2).

(112) Mr. E. K——. Aet. 28. Came on account of slight conjunctivitis. Both eyes had normal vision.

In the left eye the ophthalmoscope showed an ovoid disc, seen best with —.5 D. It had a transverse, oval cup, from the inner edge of which sprang the vessels, and also a rather broad dark-gray strand. This strand passed forward and slightly up, with a gentle curve. At this point, seen best with + 4. D., it turned sharply downward.

Farther forward, at a point seen best with + 8. D., it sent off a large number of the finest filaments, in all directions, but mainly diverging forward. In this neighborhood, and seen best with + 9½ D., was a free body in the vitreous. It consisted of two little bodies, with attached filaments joined by a twisted center fiber. The strand itself, much narrowed, continued downward and forward, its end being best seen with + 13. D. It terminated in a double knob-like enlargement, the smaller resting upon the larger.

At the inner border of the disc was a small pigment spot, and lying a short distance inward from it was another large pigment patch in the retina.

Downward from the disc was a coloboma of the choroid. Its upper edge was about a half disc-diameter from the lower edge of the disc. It was about 2 disc-diameters wide, and about 3 long. Its floor was seen best with — 1.50 D. It presented two zones; an outer one, dark-gray, with much pigment and several blood-vessels; a central area, with a few pigment spots, and two large vessels crossing it. There was a corresponding defect in the field of vision.

Remainder of the fundus and macular region normal.

At the posterior pole of the lens was attached a fine, gray filament, which passed a short distance back into the vitreous. It undulated gently on moving the eye. ▶

LORING (b)—

(113) The only case this author had seen. It was in the eye of a young adult.

The remains of the vessel had the appearance of a fine, dark-colored string, which was attached to the central part of the disc. It tapered gradually forward, terminating in a small flattened projection, not unlike the head of a serpent, by which it had evidently been attached to the posterior surface of the lens in the embryonic state.

On the posterior surface of the lens was a small, dark opacity, the point of its original attachment.

Its appearance was that of an obliterated vessel.

HASBROUCK—

(114) Lady in middle life. Left eye is highly myopic, with — 10 D., V being only equal to seeing large objects. On the posterior surface of the lens was a small opacity at the pole. No remnant of the artery was to be detected passing back from this point ; but a dark wavy cord passed forward from the region of the disc into the vitreous.

LAURENCE—

(115) Christina C——. Aet. 12 Complained of very poor vision in the right eye. Read with difficulty Jaeger No. 20. (Left, Jaeger No. 1 at ordinary distance). Ophthalmoscope showed in the R. eye a grayish, irregularly knotted, thread-like strand, attached by an enlarged, funnel-shaped, semi-transparent expansion to the central and lower part of the optic disc. Its anterior extremity was narrowed, and floated freely in the vitreous.

On the posterior aspect of the lens was a small, central opaque speck—the point of the former attachment of the hyaloid artery.

The choroid was considerably atrophied, and the refraction of the eye was myopic.

UNTERHARNSCHEIDT—

(116) Boy of 14 years, in the third grade of the gymnasium, when seen three years previous. Had then a myopia of $\frac{1}{2}$, and corrected V = $\frac{3}{4}$. Media clear.

In the left eye the ophthalmoscope showed a dark, round strand running forward through the center of the vitreous. It sprang from the large arterial branch passing upward on the disc, and was of the same caliber. It became gradually thinner, so that in the center of the vitreous it was but a fine thread; then it grew gradually thicker, and was inserted at the posterior pole of the lens by a conical base. Lens was clear. This cord was taunt, and not curved, and on movements of the eye only moved very slightly.

Three years later again seen. Myopia had increased to $\frac{1}{2}$ (an axial elongation of about $\frac{3}{4}$ mm.), and the myopic crescent had become a circular staphyloma.

The hyaloid remain had parted at the thinned central part. The portion that remained attached to the disc made wide and rapid undulations on moving the eye, showing the posterior portion of the vitreous to be fluid. The anterior portion attached to the lens was shorter, and moved but slightly.

The floating ends produced entoptic shadows, which were stated to have come on suddenly after a prolonged and severe use of the eyes in studying. To this end no doubt the increase in the axial length of the eye, and the tension upon the optic nerve, in extreme forced convergence, both contributed.

GROUP G—STRAND PASSING FROM DISC TO LENS.

This group is, next to Group E, the largest subdivision of the ordinary form.

Here the hyaloid remnant retains its attachment at its point of origin upon the disc, and as well its distal attachment at or near the posterior pole of the lens.

This and Group H are to be regarded as the groups presenting the *type form* of this anomaly, from which type all the other groups are variations, departing more or less widely.

This group contains the case reported by Saemisch, which is of interest as being the first case *put upon record*, where this anomaly was observed by the ophthalmoscope.

Debierre's case (67), shown in profile in Plate 12, Fig. 9, is a very good illustration of this group; not perfectly characteristic owing only to the unusual ending at the disc and lens.

WALLMANN—

(117) Child. Aet. 4. Died of tuberculosis. The two eyes presented examples of cystic coloboma (as is now termed).

In the left eye was an iris-coloboma, choroid-coloboma, and cystic enlargement below, as is usually found in these cases. The len is uneven, with thickened capsule. From its posterior surface there passes back a strong, gleaming white, connective tissue band, 2 mm. in width. This broadens out into a stellate shaped plate or mass, to be spread out in front of the disc; some stray fibers going to the margin of the cyst-sac below.

(118) In the right eye the same appearance was presented, only the strand is shorter and narrower, and passes back below the disc to go more directly to the cyst-margin.

SAEMISCH (a)—

(119) Miss C——. Aet. 17. Came on account of asthenopia. Had a Hm. of $\frac{1}{16}$ and the corrected V = normal.

In the left eye the ophthalmoscope showed a dark gray strand running through the vitreous from the posterior pole of the lens to the optic disc. This strand was of the diameter of a primary branch of the central vein. It consisted of an opaque central shaft which appeared almost black, and of a more transparent sheath surrounding this and looking like a gray band on all sides. The insertion on the disc was in the lower-inner quadrant; from here it passed perfectly straight through the center of the vitreous, and inserted itself into the posterior capsule by a small knob-like termination, lying just down and in from the posterior pole.

The media were perfectly clear, and the fundus normal.

ZEHENDER (b)—

(120) (Case reported to Z. by Dr. Toussaint.) Soldier. 21 years of age. Complained of poor vision and shadows before his eyes. Myopia was present,

but vitreous clear. The ophthalmoscope showed in his right eye a dark thin strand springing from the optic disc, just up and out from the point of exit of the central artery. This passed forward, gradually increasing in size for the first third of its length, like a slender goblet. It then divided into three fine branches, of which the middle one was the stronger and showed a double contour. These passed forward to be inserted into the outer quadrant of the posterior capsule. The point of their attachment was marked by a faint steel-gray opacity. The fundus was normal.

WECKER (a)—

(121) Young woman of 25 yrs. of age. Came for some lachrymal trouble Patient had always been amblyopic in the right eye. Never any injury.

On examination a delicate, translucent membrane was found stretched across the eyeball, back of the pupil. This presented an oval opening in the center, through which the fundus could be clearly seen. In the extreme upper-outer quadrant behind the iris, was the dislocated cataractous lens, and about it were some chalky masses of an intense white color. All these were adherent to this membrane (probably the anterior hyaloid). The ophthalmoscope showed a dark strand of about the diameter of a primary branch of the central artery, springing from the center of the disc at the point of exit of the vessels. It passed forward perfectly straight, rounded, and gradually increasing in thickness, to be inserted among these chalky masses lying about the posterior surface of the lens. It does not undulate in movements of the eye, but is tense.

With the proper convex glasses she counts fingers at a few feet away.

GUNN—

(122) Jos. S——. Aet. 25. Left eye with strong convergent squint, and its sight had always been defective. The iris showed a marked differentiation between the outer two-thirds and the inner third, which lies posterior to and partially hid by the outer part. It movement is sluggish and confined almost to this inner band, which seems to shrink behind the outer portion.

The lens is displaced upward, showing the striations of the suspensory ligament crossing the lower half of the pupil. The lower edge of the ectopic lens revealed a peculir coloboma. The two sides or "lobules" were at a different level antero-posteriorly, and somewhat overlapped each other. Above, where the lens is single, it is cataractous.

From the bottom of the coloboma, or where the two "lobules" fuse together, there passes back a thick, opaque cord, which traversed the vitreous to be inserted at a point a trifle above the optic disc. The vitreous shows a few fine webs, and a couple of rounded dense opacities, white by reflected light.

The optic disc is surrounded by a yellowish tissue, from which bands extend out in different directions. *Above* the disc is a large bluish-white area, quite like an ordinary coloboma of the choroid, except its position.

STÖR—

(123) Fritz A——. Aet. 17. Student in the gymnasium. R. eye had myopia of 16 without complications. L. eye had myopia, central vision abolished, and peripheral vision diminished greatly. The ophthalmoscope showed a myopic crescent, and atrophic disturbance of the choroidal pigment from the disc out to the equator. It also revealed a persistent (obliterated) hyaloid artery.

HIRSCHBERG (a)—

(124) Mr. L——. Adult. Vision was normal in right eye. L. eye J. No. 3. Left eye shows a small posterior capsular cataract. From this projects backward a broad, conical process, which appears white by oblique illumination. This passes into a thin tubular membrane, which passes back in a sinuous course through the vitreous. It tapers to a fine fiber, which is inserted into the only faintly outlined disc. Below this disc lie numerous, irregular black pigment clumps. A few pigment specks lie in front of the level of the retinal vessels. Another clump lies above toward the periphery.

MCHARDY (a)—

(125) Woman. Aet. 33. Troubled with asthenopia, due to hypermetropia. Right eye showed a filamentous, opaque band, extending from the center of the disc to the posterior pole of the lens. The band appeared white or black according to the method of illumination, and was destitute of blood. It was not tightly stretched, its center showing a slow, floating motion on rapid movements of the eye. The lens was clear every-where, except just at the point of insertion. Patient was not troubled with the entoptic phenomena, and V was $\frac{6}{5}$.

——— —(b)

(126) The author has seen another very similar case since. The persistent vessel was in the right eye, and extended as a continuous, opaque filament from the posterior pole of the lens to the optic disc. It was finely attenuated at its two attached extremities, and thicker in the middle. It floated about on movements of the eye.

There were old patches of choroido-retinal change, evidently due to hereditary syphilis.

BADAL—

(127) Patient, a woman, who presented on account of small congenital dermoid tumors at the sclero-corneal junction—three in each eye—a remarkable symmetry.

In the left eye the ophthalmoscope shows a dark opaque strand arising from the center of the disc. It passes straight forward, and is attached to the posterior pole of the lens.

It was not movable on movements of the eyeball.

LARSEN—

(128) Man. Aet. 56. Came on account of a perforating injury by a percussion cap. The ophthalmoscope revealed a small fragment of the cap, imbedded in the fundus in the neighborhood of the macula. In addition it showed a white strand springing from the disc. This passed forward through the vitreous, divided at an acute angle into two branches, which were attached to the posterior capsule of the lens.

——— —

(129) Boy. Aet. 6 years. Had congenital cataract, for which the needle operation was made. After absorption a grayish-white strand was found passing from the posterior capsule of the lens back to the optic disc. When near the disc it spread out into a club-shaped base, which covered the point of exit of the vessels.

A small coloboma of the choroid was also detected.

The other eye was normal.

REUSS—

(130) Franz Str——. Aet. 15. Patient in the surgical ward, and used as a "normal" fundus for the beginners in the ophthalmoscopic course.

The following condition was discovered: The lower-inner arterial branch was bounded by broad, white, connective tissue contours. From this branch, at the edge of the deep, sharply bounded central cup, sprang a grayish strand about the diameter of a medium vein. It passed forward; gradually thinned to a fine fibrilla; this continued in a long, bow-like curve forward to the lower-inner quadrant of the lens capsule, where it attached itself by a sharp, darkly pigmented point. It had a grayish, translucent shimmer, and oscillated distinctly on movements of the eye. Vitreous was clear, fundus normal, and refraction hypermetropic.

SNELL—

(131) Chas. R. S——. Aet. 11. Brought on account of defective vision in the right eye. Slight divergence, and V = counting fingers at one foot. Myopia of about 8 D.

At the posterior pole was an opacity made up of fine striæ. (S. compares it to the cut in Gardiner's case.) Running back from this was a light gray translucent cord, which, on direct examination, was seen as a hollow tube. This passed backward through the vitreous; at the disc widened somewhat like a funnel; and was connected with a vessel at the center of the papilla. It made free excursions on movements of the eye. It did not appear to contain blood.

RUMSZEWICZ—

This author reports two cases, with special reference to the fact that the presence of this anomaly may have no deleterious effect upon vision.

(132) CASE 1. V was $\frac{20}{40}$. The ophthalmoscope revealed a nearly transparent strand springing from the disc. It passed forward through the vitreous, to be attached to the lower part of the posterior lens capsule. Although it floated about freely upon every movement of the eye, the patient was hardly conscious of any shadows caused by it.

(133) CASE 2. In this patient V was also $\frac{20}{40}$. This strand, however, was much more distinct, being 1 mm. in width. It was black by reflected light, and very freely movable. No scotoma could be detected, and only when the patient gazed at some bright surface was he conscious of the shadows caused by it.

LITTLE—

(134) Miss W——. Aet. 20. Patient troubled with asthenopia, compelling her to cease work. V impaired, with concentric contraction of the visual field.

Right eye V $\frac{7}{200}$, with + 48c 90°. V = $\frac{20}{40}$. Ophthalmoscope shows remains of the hyaloid artery springing from the optic disc, pushing directly forward, and being attached to the posterior pole of the lens. This strand is well-marked, with dark contour at the middle of its course in the vitreous, and here probably a remnant of the vessel itself is present. At both extremities it thins out into a very delicate tracery, probably only the adventitia of the vessel, which shows like dark lace-work against the red background of the fundus. The film oscillates on movements of the globe. In the left eye was also found a small remnant of the hyaloid. (See case 16.)

VASSAUX—(Plate I, Figs. 1, 4, 5 and 6).

(135) Infant, Ed. F——. Aet. 54 days. Brought by the parents on account of the bright reflection from the left pupil, and the evident blindness of this eye. The child was healthy and well developed.

The cornea was clear; the anterior chamber was shallow; the pupil dilated irregularly under atropine, with numerous filaments from its anterior face to the front of the lens (persistent pupillary membrane); it gave back a bright yellow reflex: the lens was clear; back of it was an apparently solid surface, showing numerous small blood-vessels ramifying upon it, and the tension was increased. The diagnosis of glioma was made, and the eye was enucleated.

After hardening, the globe was divided. It presented a fine, round strand running from the center of the disc to the posterior pole of the lens. Under the microscope this proved to be a small artery enveloped in a delicate sheath. On the posterior surface of the lens was a deposit or layer spreading out in all directions from the point of insertion of the hyaloid artery. This layer is composed of fibrous tissue, separated by amorphous matrix. It contains small blood-vessels, calcareous points, and minute fat globules. To all sides the elongated ciliary processes are fused with this layer. This is no doubt a remnant of the post-capsular membrane, thickened and opaque. It was its presence which led to the error in diagnosis.

SATTLER—

(136) Patient came to Professor Arlt's clinic to be operated for cataract. An opaque layer upon the posterior capsule was so dense that nothing could be seen of the vitreous chamber and fundus. The needle operation was repeatedly made, and fair vision was given. The posterior polar cataract was not absorbed, but pushed to one side, the patient seeing past it. Examination showed a persistent hyaloid artery, previously concealed from view.

GALEZOWSKI—

(137-8) This author adds two cases of persistent hyaloid artery of the ordinary type, occurring in the form of an opaque fibrous strand, with the two ends fixed, the one at the papilla, and the other at the posterior surface of the lens. The vessel itself obliterated.

In one case the lenticular attachment was the seat of a posterior capsular cataract.

NETTLESHIP—

(139) Emma G——-. Aet. 5. Child was brought on account of trouble in the left eye. The cornea was steamy, the pupil dilated, and gave back a yellowish reflex. Fearing malignant growth, the eye was enucleated by Hutchinson. The eyeball was hardened and opened. The vitreous chamber was filled with a soft, granular, altered vitreous. Washing this away, two strands were found traversing the vitreous. One was about the size of a strong sewing thread, the other more delicate. They were close together, attached behind with an expanded foot about 2.5 mm. to the inner side of the optic disc, which was hid by fibrous tissue, probably thickened hyaloid membrane; and attached in front by a similar expansion at about the middle of the posterior lens-capsule. They were stretched taut and stiff. There were some fine striæ, and much rust-colored pigment in the anterior part of the vitreous.

On microscopic examination the larger strand was found to contain *two* large blood-vessels running through its entire length. They took origin from one or two of the large retinal vessels at the expanded base of the cord. At the back of the lens they divided into branches which were traced only a short distance, and whose mode of ending was not ascertained. The smaller cord contained no blood-vessel.

The cords were composed of reticulated fibrous tissue, with round or oval cells in the meshes. This tissue was loose and open around the vessel, and more compact at the outer layer.

In front the cords expanded and joined a fibrous layer at the back of the lens, which layer was continued laterally into the thickened hyaloid covering the ciliary body. The entire retina seemed thickened, which in fact was due to a general thickening of the hyaloid membrane; which thickening was most marked at the posterior pole, where the expanded base of the strands passed into it. Just at this point there were numerous blood-vessels, although the rest of this thickened tissue contained comparatively few. There were numerous microscopical changes in almost all the intra-ocular structures, not necessary here to specify; the interesting point is, that this keen observer is of the opinion that the entire abnormal series started from this persistent hyaloid vessel, and the nutritive disturbances it initiated.

BRAILEY—

(140) John A. D——. Aet. 15. Two years before, the left eye had been injured by the bounding recoil of a toy cannon.

Eye is congested, somewhat painful and no P. L. Enucleated by Mr. Critchett. Cornea clear; iris only a rim, and adherent to the lens; choroid mottled near the disc; and retina detached into a funnel-shaped column in the axis of the vitreous. In the center of this funnel, extending forward from the disc, is a tough fibrous cord. It runs forward about a quarter of an inch and bifurcates. The outer branch runs forward, is flattened out over the outer quadrant of the posterior lens capsule, and blends with it. The inner branch is similarly distributed, but a tough bands runs from it to just behind the ciliary processes and ends. The cord and its branches are closely wrapped by the detached retina.

This cord consists of indistinct white fibrous tissue, along the center of which runs a more marked band of fibers, in which a few scattered pigment particles are found.

BECKER (b)—

(141) Patient was a man operated on for cataract in the left eye. In the right eye he had quite well marked microphthalmus. Vision was reduced to counting fingers at a few feet, and was not improved by glasses. The iris was crater-like and pupil small, but it could be dilated with atropine sufficiently to show the fundus. The lens was situated well back in the vitreous, and was fixed in place by a persistent pupillary membrane in front, and behind by a persistent hyaloid artery running from it to the disc. There was a so-called coloboma of the nerve. There was no coloboma of the choroid, and no defect of the visual field.

(Prof. Becker had observed this sort of remnant on three other occasions, when dissecting microphthalmic eyeballs.)

Manz (a)—(Plate I, Fig. 3, and Plate XII, Fig. 6).

(142) An anencephalic fœtus, almost (or quite) at full term, 38 cm. (about 15 in.) in length.

At the center of the disc was found a conical process occupying the porus opticus. This was 1-2 mm. in length, and was composed of a blood-vessel surrounded by a cellular envelope (Plate 1, Fig. 3). This cellular sheath ended at the level of the retina. The obliterated blood-vessel, surrounded by a well-marked adventitia, passed forward through the vitreous. It soon divided into two branches; one passed forward to the center of the posterior capsule; the other, when close to the lens, turned aside and passed to the ciliary body.

(In all eight examples of anencephalus that he examined, a hyaloid artery was found present; but, as most of these were in the earlier months, this was to be anticipated.)

Wedl and Bock—

(143) These authors give an illustration in their Atlas of a persistent hyaloid artery, from an eye in the collection of Prof. Stellwag.

The strand traverses the vitreous from the disc to the posterior capsule of the lens. Only in its anterior portions were found remnants of the blood-vessel. At this point there were also cell-proliferation in the surrounding tissue.

(This example came to my attention too late to be utilized in our Plates 1 or 12, and I can only refer my readers to the original.)

Group H—Persistent Vessels containing Blood.

This group forms a small one, really a sub-group to that preceeding it, Group G; but these cases are of such special interest that it seems best to place them in a group by themselves.

The cases reported by Gardiner, Eversbusch, and Tangeman are of particular interest, as here the vessel and its branches, carrying blood, remain practically in the very same stage as they existed during their activity in the embryonic condition.

In the older cases of Zehender and Liebreich it is difficult to imagine what became of the blood when it reached the posterior pole of the perfectly transparent lens. Possibly some extremely delicate capillaries, invisible to the ophthalmoscope and naked eye, carried it away. In the more recent cases, that have been much more carefully observed, like those of Eversbusch, Gardiner, Tangeman, etc., these terminal vessels were seen, spreading out to go to the ciliary region, and so carry off the blood.

In the cases that have been examined microscopically, like those of Vassaux, Haab, Hess, etc., this termination of the vessels was clearly made out. Of course, this arrangement was to be assumed, *a priori*, for no other arrangement seems supposable under the circumstances, and from the facts of development.

The case of Tangeman (147), shown in profile in Plate 12, Fig. 8, is probably the most characteristic example of this group.

There is quite a group of cases that have usually been included under the head of persistent hyaloid vessels, which, if included here, would swell this group to very considerable proportions. These are the cases where a vessel containing blood emerges from the disc, passes a greater or less distance forward into the vitreous, and then turns upon itself to pass back again to the disc or retina. It either disappears in the disc, or is distributed to the retina.

The following cases are either frequently quoted, or are found on examination to belong to this class:

> Liebreich—Trans. Path. Soc'y. London, 1871.
> Little—Trans. Amer. Ophth. Soc'y. (17th.) 1875.
> Schrapinger—Arch. Ophth. and Otol. III. 1873.
> Czermak—Centralbl. für Augenh'de. VII. 1883.
> Reibau—Charitè Annalen. I. 1876.
> Fournet—Recueil d'Ophthalmologie. II. 1880.
> Hirschberg—Centralb. für Augenh'l'de. 5, 7, and 9. 1881-3-5.
> Callan (2 cases)—N. Y. Med. Jl. XXII. 1875.
> Kipp—(Left eye of his case—109.)
> Szili—Centralbl. für Augenh'l'de. IX. 1885.
> Hunike—Amer. Jour. of Ophthal. II. 1885.
> Frost—Trans. Ophth. Soc., United King. VII. 1887.
>   —and a number of others.

It is manifestly erroneous to include these cases under the head of persistent hyaloid vessels. They have no genetic claim here. Only the most superficial consideration, misled by position alone, can regard them as belonging here. Until their more detailed consideration in another chapter, they may be regarded as anomalous branches of the arteria centralis retinæ.

In connection with this Group H, refer to the cases of Königstein (46), Kipp (109), and Nettleship (139), where the strand, or a portion of it, contains blood.

ZEHENDER (*a*)—

   (144) Adult, man. Seen in 1857 in the Rostock Surgical Clinic. The ophthalmoscope showed a curved strand running through the axis of the vitreous. It sprang from the center of the disc with the central vessels, and for a short distance this posterior extremity showed red like the other vessels. It passed forward to terminate in a knob-like, flattened anterior extremity, attached to the posterior capsule a trifle to the outer side of the posterior pole. This attachment was irregularly circular, with several short, blunt, rounded processes, and gave a good light reflex. The strand, in its central portions, appeared dark, with the ophthalmoscope. With the oblique illumination the anterior portion of the strand, so far as it could be followed

back, presented a blood-red color. The strand showed snake-like undulations on movements of the globe. There was no doubt of the vessel being still open, and its lumen filled with blood.

LIEBREICH—

(145) (Case reported to Professor Zehender.) Here there was a wide and deep physiological cup. From the central artery in the cup there sprang forward a small branch, filled with blood. This passed forward a short distance, rapidly narrowed, and was continued forward as a thin, gray strand. This passed to the posterior capsule, and was attached by a star-shaped, white clump.

The fine strand was straight, and did not undulate on movement of the globe.

BAYER (a)—(Plate XI, Fig. 2).

(146) Marie T——. Aet. 14. Has V practically nil in the left eye, with nystagmus and strabismus convergens. The right eye has also poor vision.

The ophthalmoscope showed a curious anomaly of the disc. It is a semicircular, atropic disc, with its lower, straight margin nearly horizontal. From this lower margin spring all the vessels; three passing down, and two passing across the disc and being distributed above.

From this lower margin, at its center, there springs also a strand, which passes into the vitreous. Its center is dark, cord-like and red, and this is surrounded by a delicate gray sheath. Anteriorly this becomes funnel-shaped, and spreads out over a gray, angular plate, which lies in the upper-outer part of the anterior vitreous. This sends processes upward. Here also the red axis can be observed—showing that the vessel continues forward to the posterior capsule of the lens.

This strand undulates on movements of the eye.

To the outer side of the disc there is a large, vertical, obelisk-shaped area of congenital choroiditis. This presents a few patches of a white, gleaming ground. Over this run some few small vessels, and in it are numerous black pigment masses and dark red-brown plaques.

TANGEMAN—

(147) Patient an adult. Came for treatment of granular conjunctivitis, both eyes. Vision was normal in the left eye, and $\frac{20}{100}$ in the right. The vision in this eye had been " blurred " as long as he could remember.

An ophthalmoscopic examination of the right eye showed lens and vitreous clear, and the papilla and fundus normal. From the central artery upon the disc one large vessel passed forward through the center of the vitreous. When one-third the distance to the lens, it divided at a very acute angle into two smaller branches, which continued forward, only slightly diverging. Just behind the lens these two again divide dichotomously; and these secondary branches, passing to the posterior surface of the lens capsule, broke up into a large number (15–20) of minute branches, which radiated toward the periphery, to be lost to view even with the pupil dilated ad maximum. All these vessels were bright red, carrying arterial blood. This was distinct and unquestionable, for all the media were perfectly transparent.

GARDINER—

(148) T. N——. Aet. 22. Came on account of dimness of sight.

Ophthalmoscopic examination showed floating opacities in the vitreous in the left eye. In the right eye it revealed a white, shining cord running through the center of the vitreous from the optic disc to the posterior pole of the lens.

At its posterior end it began as a funnel-shaped expansion, entirely covering the papilla and its vessels, and extending a little beyond it at the nasal side. The trunk was straight and about the diameter of one of the principal branches of the retinal artery. This cord in the erect image, exhibited rhythmic movements, and was seen to be formed of a bright and central blood-vessel, enveloped in a thin, translucent sheath. At its anterior end it spread into a similar, but smaller, funnel-shaped expansion, which was attached to the posterior capsule of the lens. This expansion on the posterior capsule, examined with a strong convex lens, is seen to be composed of numerous little blood-vessels radiating and ramifying over the polar region of the posterior capsule. The vitreous was somewhat hazy. V $= \frac{20}{200}$.

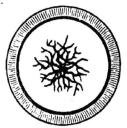

FIG. 4.

This cut is the only one I know illustrating these post-capsular vessels remaining in the living subject. They here are shown very tortuous, and almost as if they anastomose. How much of this is due to artist and engraver I can not say. In Kölliker's injections of the fœtal eye these vessels pass almost straight from the pole to the periphery; and in my cases (Plate XII, Figs. 1 and 2) this condition is also very clearly shown.

In the cases of Vassaux and Haab, a similar tortuous condition is shown; but here there had been pathological changes to account for it.

HAAB—(Plate XII, Fig. 5, and Plate I, Fig. 2).

(149) Heinrich K——. Aet. 5. The little patient had presented hydrophthalmus congenitus of the right eye. When but a few months old, his case had been described by Muralt ("Hydrophthalmus congenitus," Inaug. Diss., Zurich, 1869, p. 47). At 5 years of age his eye had been enucleated by Horner, and the divided globe figured by Becker: ("Photographische Abbildungen von Durchschnitten gesunder und kranker Augen," Series II, No. 20.)

The anterior aspect of the vitreous was closed in by a partition composed of the suspensory ligament, and the shrunken, plate-like lens. From the center of this there projected backward a rounded strand 4.5 mm. in length. This was supposed to be the remnant of the hyaloid artery. Under the microscope this was demonstrated to be a blood-vessel, and as its lumen was still filled with blood it was inferred that it was a portion only of the open artery that had passed back to connect with the central artery, and which had been torn away in removing the vitreous after long hardening in alcohol.

EVERSBUSCH (b)—

(150) Child a few days old sent for examination. Had coloboma of the iris, downward in each eye.

In the iris clefts, could be made out a white triangular process. This filled up the floor of the coloboma, and passed back in contact with the inferior edge of the lens.

With the ophthalmoscope the vitreous is seen to be traversed by a blood-vessel (red in color), which makes free excursions on movements of the globe. Back of the lens this breaks up into a number of terminal branches which pass to this process lying below. This process is seen to be continued back into a broad gray mass, which covers the floor of the vitreous chamber and passes up to hide the disc. The hyaloid artery is seen to disappear posteriorly in this mass.

A few weeks later the child died of pneumonia. On making sections of the eye, the hyaloid artery was traced directly into the arteria centralis retinæ. The gray mass was traced directly into the sclera below, and was found to be identical with it in histological structure. It was no doubt a remnant of the earlier mesoderm process.

HESS—

(151) Child. Aet. 3 weeks. The left eye presented an examples of microphthalmus, being but 10 mm. in diameter (the right was normal). The child dying from lung trouble, an opportunity to examine the eye was given.

From the optic disc there passed forward a strand fully as thick as the nerve itself. This was composed of a very large hyaloid artery, whose adventitia and muscular coats were very beautifully developed. This was surrounded by a sheath of rather loose tissue, showing numerous round and a few spindle-shaped cells. This sheath was of conical shape, becoming narrower as it passed forward, until at the middle of the vitreous it was reduced to a very thin band.

From here the strand again widened funnel-like, to finally spread out into a thick membrane covering almost the entire posterior capsule of the lens. In this membrane the artery broke up into a large number of fine branches. The membrane was made up of spindle-shaped cells with oval nuclei. The lens itself is small, being but 4 mm. in diameter; and is displaced upward to an extent that almost brings its lower margin in the anterior-posterior axis of the globe.

A strong bundle of this hyaloid strand is continued around the lower margin of the lens, passes forward and downward through a coloboma of the iris, which is present at the usual site, and divides into two bundles, a thin bundle, containing delicate vessels passing around upon the anterior capsule and becoming joined with the iris, and a thicker bundle passing to the region of the canals of Fontana, blending with the sclera and choroid.

The iris and ciliary processes above are adherent to the anterior face of the lens; below they turn back along the lower surface of the bundle which passes forward through the coloboma.

This case has a great resemblance to the one above, as regards this band passing forward through the coloboma; and both cases will afford us further study, when the question of coloboma of the iris and choroid is taken up.

GROUP I—STRAND ATTACHED TO THE LENS ALONE.

This group includes a few cases in which the only vestige of the hyaloid artery is a filament attached to the posterior pole of the lens, projecting back and ending free and movable in the vitreous. The disc is in all the cases perfectly free. The fundus is normal, and the vitreous clear.

In 1880, at the time I saw Dr. Seely's case (154), we imagined that this was a unique case; but careful seach reveals a few published prior to this, and a few have been published since. Ammon's case, figured in Plate I, Fig. 7, is the earliest, and one of the most typical. Of course it was only discovered post-mortem.

This cut, which was the one used to illustrate Dr. Seely's case, and is kindly loaned by the secretary of the American Ophthalmological Society, shows the condition in this group as well as any. An ophthalmoscopic picture is not practicable.

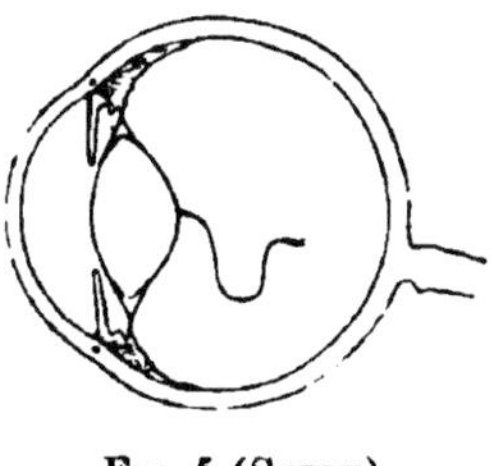

FIG. 5 (SEELY).

A few cases in the other groups present little filaments projecting from the posterior pole of the lens; which if occurring alone would bring them under this group.

AMMON (a)—(Plate I, Fig. 7).

(152) This auther figures in his large Atlas a lens which presents several congenital anomalies. From its posterior pole there projects a short, but well-marked remnant of the hyaloid artery; in line with this is a narrow, rounded axial cataract, and at the center of the lens this broadens into a small, not well-marked nuclear cataract.

The entire lens shows an anomalous bulging back of the posterior portion—a case of lenticonus posterior.

SAEMISCH (b)—

(153) Mrs. D——. Aet. 60. Came on account of failing vision. A beginning cortical cataract was found, but not so much developed but that the fundus could be clearly seen. The ophthalmoscope showed a dark, opaque clump at the posterior pole (the adjacent lens still clear). From this there passed back a gray strand about the thickness of a primary branch of the central artery. This did not reach the disc, but its somewhat frayed-out end drooped downward—however it would have reached the disc apparently had it been stretched out straight. On moving the eyeball this posterior extremity made wide and free excursions; while the anterior two-thirds undulated but slightly.

The vitreous was clear, the fundus normal, and the disc perfectly free from any remains.

SEELY—

(154) John V. V——. Aet. 30. Student at the Medical College of Ohio. Practicing physicion, now in Kentucky. Had noticed dimness of vision in his left eye for eighteen years past. V was $\frac{20}{200}$, and with either $+ 1.50c\ 90°$, or $— 1.50c\ 180°$, V $= \frac{20}{78}$.

The mirror revealed a dark, brownish, thread-like strand attached at the exact posterior pole of the lens. Its point of attachment was marked by a very small conical base. It floated free in the fluidified vitreous, making extensive vermicular oscillations on movement of the eye; but always coming to rest in a dependent position, curving toward the floor of the vitreous chamber. At times, when it would shoot backward, it seemed nearly if not quite long enough to reach to the disc.

The ophthalmoscope showed a clear disc, with no trace of its previous attachment at this point.

The wood-cut is from a drawing of my own, Dr. Seely kindly calling me in to examine the case with him.

WEBSTER—

(155) Miss M. H——. Aet. 22. Came on account of a blow received on the eye. Refraction, E. and V $= \frac{20}{78}$. No previous eye trouble.

Ophthalmoscope revealed in the left eye a filamentous body in the vitreous. It was attached anteriorly by a conical base to the posterior capsule of the lens, about one line to the nasal side of the posterior pole.

It passed back as a dark, solid, cylindrical strand of uniform size, and about the diameter of one of the primary branches of the arteria centralis. Its posterior extremity dwindled to a point which was *fixed* in the vitreous about 2 mm. in front of the retinal level, and just above and to the nasal side of the disc, in front of a retinal vein. Possibly it was fixed in this position by a fine extension too transparent to be seen, which passed to this vein, or to the adjacent retina or disc.

On movement of the eye it showed wave-like undulations, like a loose rope, attached at its two ends, and shaken.

RIGHT EYE.—There was a small filament lying just back of the posterior capsule, to the nasal side of the posterior pole. It made extremely limited excursions on any movements of the eye, showing that it was not fixed to the posterior capsule, but was probably loosely attached to it by a delicate film, too transparent to be visible by the ophthalmoscope or oblique illumination.

HASBROUCK—

(156) T——. Aet. 15. Boy had my. ast., and with proper correction had normal V in R. eye and $\frac{5}{7}$ in L. eye. In this eye the rudiment of the hyaloid artery was attached at the posterior pole of the lens, and extended well back into the vitreous. It waved about with a vermicular movement on all movements of the eyeball.

The disc was normal, with the physiological cup much deeper even than in the other eye.

One year later V had become $\frac{5}{6}$.

REUSS—

(157) Adolf R——. Aet. 15. Left eye has V $= \frac{6}{36}$; with $+ 2.50$, V $= \frac{6}{17}$. Remains of the hyaloid are present. The disc is clear, and shows no trace of

the original attachment. It has a small underlying conus. Some distance in front of the disc commences a bluish-white, transparent sheath, much like a wall to the central canal of the vitreous. Within this sheath is plainly visible a more solid, bluish strand, whose inner contour is sharp and straight, but whose temporal edge is uneven and thrown into minute folds, somewhat like a feather-edge.

This central strand is short, and sends one very short, thick branch downward. Its anterior end is blunt and slightly knobbed, and does not reach to the posterior surface of the lens.

At the posterior pole is a small, opaque spot, from which passes back a translucent, thin fiber. This curves backward in a corkscrew-like manner, not directly toward the central strand. It, however, soon bends in a whip-like manner toward this strand, and seems to join or wind about its blunt anterior end.

(This patient is the same whose right eye is described in case 61.)

Meyer—

(158) Karl E——. Aet. 10. Case was one from the private practice of Professor Becker (Heidelberg). The boy presented the rare anomaly, lenticonus posterior, in the right eye. From the posterior surface of the lens bulged back a well-marked conical process. This was transparent, except exactly at its apex was a dense white opacity, about 5 mm. long and half as wide, which was bordered around half its periphery by a sharp, dark line close to and parallel with its border. Inward from this was another white opacity about half this size; and scattered about these were a number of minute, point-like opacities. The lenticonus was inclosed by a delicate, membranous funnel or conical sheath ("Kegelmantel"), which had its base attached to the posterior surface of the lens. This sheath projected far back into the vitreous, in the axis of the globe. It reflected the light strongly, although very delicate in texture.

The V was reduced to counting fingers at 3–4 meters; claimed to see better with − 12 D., but was not really improved. Fundus was normal. By the direct method, the speck at the apex of the posterior pole could be most clearly seen with + 28 D.

Meyer seems puzzled to account for the genesis of such a case; but the central posterior capsular cataract, and the tubular sheath, which can be nothing else than a persistent portion of the hyaloid canal, seem to clearly place the case here. Compare the case of Ammon (No. 152), figured on Plate 1, Fig. 7, and the cases of Oeller (163) and those in Group L.

Kipp (b)—

(159) Girl. Aet. 16. She had always been troubled with linear shadows crossing the field of vision—in the left eye.

The ophthalmoscope revealed a dark-colored, thread-like strand in the vitreous. It was apparently attached to the posterior pole of the lens, extended back into the vitreous, where it ended free. It floated about readily on any movement of the eye, occasioning the entoptic phenomena mentioned above.

The media and fundus were otherwise normal, but V was only $\frac{6}{36}$. In the right eye, V = $\frac{6}{5}$

Group J—Posterior Capsular Cataract.

The cases where an opacity exists at the posterior pole of the lens may be divided into several groups. A certain number of these cases are acquired forms, secondary to inflammatory trouble in the vitreous, ciliary body, choroid, etc., and these may be set aside at once. The remainder are congenital. These congenital forms are probably *all* due *primarily* to a disturbance occasioned by the presence and subsequent obliteration of the hyaloid artery. This view was advanced long ago by Ammon, Müller, and even Himly. Oeller has more recently strongly advocated this hypothesis. Convenient classification, however, necessitates the further division of these cases. ·

In a certain number, a gray opacity exists at the posterior pole of the lens, just *beneath* the capsule. These opacities are usually stellate, with three pointed or rounded projections from the central part, forming, ordinarily, angles of about 120° with each other, and usually coinciding with the normal sector lines of the lens. For these cases it seems better to retain (and confine), the name of congenital posterior *polar* cataract. It is also more convenient to refer their extended consideration to the chapter on congenital cataract.

There remains a certain class of cases in which a rounded or irregular opacity exists *upon the posterior surface* of the posterior capsule. This is usually, but not always, situated at the posterior pole, and shows brown or dark gray. Any short processes it may send out are not arranged upon any regular plan, except that they always radiate toward the periphery of the lens. For this form it seems best to confine the name of congenital posterior *capsular* cataract. That these represent a vestige remaining at the point of lenticular attachment of the hyaloid artery is apparent, and their extended consideration may properly find a place here.

I am well aware that this is a direct reversal of the terms as used by Stellwag, but in the interests of exact nomenclature I am constrained to make it. The former group are opacities situated at the *pole* of the lens, in the lens substance, and are not necessarily connected with the capsule, *per se*. They are *polar cataracts*. The latter group are opacities upon the capsule, and need not necessarily be at the posterior pole at all. They are *capsular opacities*. So designated they are analogous to the anterior capsular or pyramidal cataracts—both due to influences extraneous to the lens itself.

Considering the not rare occurrence of all these forms of posterior lenticular opacity, it has seemed strange that so few cases illustrating this last group are to be found in the literature. It seems an instance of observers not considering it worth while to report common and well recognized forms.

The first case quoted, that of Mackenzie, is of some historic interest, for there is a probability that this is the only instance in which the persistent hyaloid remain had been observed in the living subject prior to the discovery of the ophthalmoscope.

What few cases can be recorded here illustrate very well the various forms under which this rudiment presents itself. The only form not noted is the very minute form, where a mere speck occurs at or near the posterior pole of the lens. It is almost impossible to make them out by oblique illumination, but by reflected light they show a minute black speck upon the red background. The first impression always is that we have a little foreign body upon the cornea, until the parallactic movement shows it to be back of the iris. They are extremely common, we having seen three in the current session at the College Clinic. The whole group is of common occurrence, one can hardly pick up the annual report of any clinic without finding several cases recorded.

This group is intimately connected with some of the previous ones, especially group F, where we find these posterior capsular specks present. It is also very closely connected with the following group, for we find very frequently that these posterior capsular cataracts have little striæ radiating from them. It is really difficult to decide in some of these cases whether they belong in this group or in the next. For example see Plate XII, Fig. 10.

MACKENZIE—

(160) Patient was a young man whose vision alternated frequently, at times poor, again normal (probably refractive strain). He had headaches and photopsies. "Deep in the right vitreous humor a spotted opaque appearance was observed. On dilating the pupil it was evident that there were two sets of opacities behind the lens. One, consisting of a central spot with numerous opaque threads radiating from it, especially downward and outward, was situated exactly in the axis of the eye, and a little way behind the lens [on the posterior capsule (?)]. The other opaque spot was much deeper in the eye, without any radii, and evidently moved up and down when the patient moved his eye."

This was probably either the anterior detached end of a persistent hyaloid artery, or a film attached to the posterior polar cataract. The author regarded it as hyaloiditis (?).

AMMON (b)—

(161) Girl. Aet. 3. In the left eye was present an irregular, whitish or gray opacity, situated upon the capsule at the posterior pole of the lens.

The author gives an excellent colored drawing (hard to distinguish from anterior capsular cataract, because here no perspective can be utilized in our drawings and cuts).

BERTHOLD (*b*)—

(162) Case of buphthalmus, similar to the case of Haab, presenting a posterior capsular cataract with persistence of a remnant of the hyaloid vessels. The posterior layers of the lens are finely striated and traversed by numerous small obliterated vessels. The lens is but slightly altered in form and the capsular epithelium could be traced on the anterior face.

OELLER—

(163) S. K——. Aet. 18 mos. Strong, active boy baby. Had irideremia totalis in both eyes, with rudimentary condition of the ciliary processes. Nystagmus.

The mirror shows at the posterior pole a black opacity about 1 mm. in diameter. From it radiate three fine striæ, each 1 mm. in length; one directly outward, one down and outward, one down and inward. The first two end here; the latter is continued as a fine thread-like strand toward the periphery, and bends around the lower-inner lens margin. Two mm. from the margin it divides into two fine branches, one passing upward, the other directly outward, but neither reaching the outer half of the lens. At the upper-outer border another fine strand curves over the border and passes toward the anterior pole. No connection with the posterior polar opacity could be detected, and it formed no anastomosis with the other two striæ. With the mirror these fibers appeared black, with oblique illumination as white threads. At the posterior pole there existed a little, circular, cup-like body. This surrounded the black opacity which sat in its center. This ring was about 2 mm. in diameter, and projected back into the vitreous about 2 mm. By tilting the mirror the light could be made to play first on its inner and then on its outer wall. No further rudiment of the artery was seen projecting backward; the vitreous was perfectly clear; the disc was normal, and presented no trace of any rudiment of the hyaloid artery. Similar condition existed in the other eye. Child was seen again when 5 years old, his vision was good enough to enable him to run around nicely, and play.

BERTHOLD (*a*)—

(164) Child only a few hours old, brought on account of the abnormal appearance of the eyes. The left eye was larger than the right; the cornea was oval and opaque; it was covered in its outer zone by fine vessels; and the sclera presented a dark blue ectatic zone below.

Fifteen months later this eye showed a marked exophthalmus, and the other appearances were still more exaggerated. The eye was enucleated. The lens was found flattened but transparent. The ciliary processes were adherent to its posterior surface, and reached to a round, white, firm plate (5 mm. in diameter), covering the posterior pole. This disc was readily shelled out, leaving a concave depression in the lens surface. Upon microscopic examination this little plate presented upon its anterior face, the unchanged lens capsule. The plate itself was composed of finely striated tissue, traversed by a rich plexus of embryonic blood-vessels. These formed numerous anastomoses, resulting in little star-shaped figures.

The optic papilla projected a trifle into the vitreous. Upon it was a layer of vitreous, which still contained little tufts of embryonic blood-vessels.

WILDE—

(165) M. H——. Aet 15. With impaired vision from birth.

A dense brownish-yellow opacity, circular in shape, larger in the left eye than in the right, occupied the apex of the posterior surface of the lens. Surrounding these was a slight nebulous haze, with a well-defined edge. (Good wood-cuts in the original.)

The needle operation was successfully performed, and he was able to do out-door work; but he was unable to read, and derived less aid from glasses than any case of congenital cataract that the author had met.

(166) Middle-aged man. This case presented a yellowish spot, with a few radiating fibers, very deeply situated in each lens. The lenses later became opaque, and were successfully extracted. In each there was demonstrated the opacity upon the apex of the posterior surface of the lens.

The man worked subsequently at his trade of shoemaker.

FELSER—

(167–8) Franz K——. Aet. 23. This case was one of total irideremia, and absence of the ciliary processes, both eyes.

In both lenses the posterior capsule was opaque in a peculiar and symmetrical manner. In each lens only one quadrant was left free; the upper-inner in the right eye, and the upper-outer in the left eye.

In the right eye at the posterior pole was a round opacity; this was surrounded by a narrow transparent ring, and from this radiated grayish striæ of various lengths and degrees of distinctness, in all directions toward the equator. These conditions were not present in the left eye.

Both discs were partially atrophic, dirty gray, and the arteries somewhat narrowed. $V = \frac{2}{30}$, not improved by glasses. R. eye read No. 1 at 2 in. with + 15.

DEBECK—

(169) John B——. Aet. 60. Came on account of occasional trouble with vision. The ophthalmoscope showed the lens perfectly clear. At the posterior pole on each lens was a capsular cataract. These were perfectly circular, and the same size in each eye, $2\frac{1}{4}$ mm. in diameter. They were outside the capsule, and concave, for the little posterior inverted image swept over them without appreciable change or distortion. With the mirror they showed sharply outlined, but quite thin at the edges, and became darker at the center. This would indicate a concavo-convex disc, with a distinct protrusion of the convex surface into the vitreous. It gave the impression in fact, of a nipple-like projection backward. By oblique illumination it appeared brown, and gave back a distinct reflex. His complaints of seeing poorly during the day and while at work, but better in the evening, were simply indications that at his age his pupils had become normally of about the same diameter as the round cataract. Under cocaine mydriasis his V was normal.

——— —(Plate XII, Fig. 10).

(170) James M——. Aet. 18. In the right eye presented a stellate (three rayed), posterior polar cataract. In the left eye there was a dark, thick spot at the posterior pole of the lens. From appearance it was evidently nipple-like, projecting slightly into the vitreous. From it there passed a ray upward-outward, which ended blunt; a ray upward-inward, which divided into two fine striæ; and a ray downward-inward, which also divided into two fine striæ. These striæ were not hazy streaks, but showed solid and sharply contoured.

V was not normal, but better in this eye than in the right, with its larger stellate cataract.

MÜLLER, D. E.—

(171) H. J——. Aet. 24. Strong, healthy servant girl. Has very poor vision. Left eye presents divergent strabismus, and vision only equal to poor perception of large objects. In this eye was found a zonular and axial cataract combined. In the right eye the dilated pupil revealed, at the posterior pole of the lens, a thick, sharply outlined, glittering white opacity, about the size of a hemp seed (3 to 4 mm.). From this radiated a number of fine striæ (½-1 mm. in length). In addition, 2 longer (2-3 mm.) and more distinct striæ ran downward for this distance upon the lens capsule, then turned sharply inward and faded away toward the center of the lens. Eye highly myopic, but very close vision is sharp. Reads fine print readily at 3 in.

(Two of her sisters are affected with zonular cataract.)

GROUP K—STRIÆ ON THE POSTERIOR LENS CAPSULE.

This small group includes but four reported cases, and two of my own. In these the only vestige left of the fœtal vessels which formerly ramified over the posterior surface of the growing lens, are a few white or gray striæ which cross the posterior capsule in radial lines. All other vestiges of the hyaloid system have disappeared. These striæ are thin, rounded, solid looking and sharply contoured. Although I have found but these few typical cases where the radiating striæ are the *only* vestiges remaining, a few similar cases occur among the other groups, where such striæ are found in connection with other forms, particularly in cases of posterior capsular cataract.

Frequently there is found in the calf at birth (and in a few other Mammalia), a network of vessels containing blood, which ramifies over the posterior capsule. In such cases the appearance described above is not of rare occurrence.

In the case of Gardiner (148), similar little vessels containing blood ramified over the capsule, and support the view that these striæ are such blood-vessels obliterated.

There will probably be little or no question as to this explanation of these fine striæ upon the lens capsule. Possibly some may question putting Ammon's case (Plate XII, Fig. 11), in this category. The original drawing of that case is quite unsatisfactory, and my reproduction in pen and ink necessarily quite diagrammatic. But any argument against this case on account of the remarkable regularity and artistic curves of the radiating bands, will bear just as strongly against any explanation of their origin. In my case (Plate XII, Fig. 2, L), the striæ are accurately reproduced, and bear some resemblance to Ammon's case.

WILDE—(Plate XII, Fig. 3).

(172) This author gives a wood-cut of the right eye of one of his cases. The lens is clear with the exception of three peripheral opacities; one rather large one in the lower quadrant, one small one in the upper-outer, and one in the upper-inner quadrant. There are six short striæ upon the posterior capsule, distributed around the periphery, and all reaching in about half way to the posterior pole. This author states, "we occasionally perceive a number of white lines passing out to the circumference of the lens . . . situated on the posterior surface of the lens, having their bases at the extreme edge, and their apices pointing to the center."

AMMON (Plate XII, Fig. 11).

(173) Augusta G——. Aet. 12. This girl presented irideremia totalis, both eyes. In each eye was discovered a stellate figure, deeply seated and showing a concave surface—evidently upon the posterior surface of the lens.

The rays, eight in number, begin rather faint and obscure at the posterior pole of the lens. They pass to the periphery, are somewhat curved and flame-like, and become much more distinct and sharply marked at their broader ends. The bands are distinctly striated, but the description does not so clearly indicate that they are made up of fibrous cords as to render us perfectly positive in placing this case here.

V was, of course, poor.

BERGER, E. (b)—

(174) Elizabeth B——. Aet. 12. Patient with mixed astigmatism. Corrected V = $\frac{20}{18}$.

In the R. eye the mirror and oblique illumination, revealed a white thread-like filament on the posterior lens capsule. It crossed or began at the posterior pole, and ran in quite a straight line down-outward, and up-inward. This filament was not in the lens substance, for the reflected image from the posterior lens surface was not distorted by it. No polar cataract and no filament passing back into the vitreous were present.

WEBSTER—

(175) Jas. K. W——. Aet. 24. This was an interesting case of lenticonous anterior, and is described at length.

The concluding paragraph mentions that there was also present a small posterior polar cataract, and that the whole posterior capsule was dotted over with very minute, linear opacities radiating from the posterior pole of the lens. He states that there were also delicate changes in the retina, probably congenital; but gives no description of them.

DEBECK—(Plate XII, Fig. 1, R and L.)

Bridget G——. Aet. 44. Came on account of beginning presbyopia. With + 1.00, V = $\frac{20}{18}$, each eye. With + 2.00, J No. 2 fairly well. With the mirror a number of fine dark strands were detected on the lower segment of the capsule in each eye. By the oblique illumination these were clearly seen to be fine, distinctly rounded, white or light gray fibers, of sharp contour.

(176) In the right eye one started from the posterior pole, soon divided, and one of the branches again divided. The other six were peripheral, and two of these divided.

(177) In the left eye, one started from near the pole, and further out divided; the other five were peripheral and single. By maximum atropine dilatation these could not be traced beyond the lens border. The lens was absolutely clear, the vitreous and fundus normal, and no vestige could be detected upon the disc.

DeBeck—(Plate XII, Fig. 2, R. and L.).

Jas. H. T——. Aet. 34. The colored porter in the office of the Addyston Pipe and Steel Works. Came on account of poor vision and asthenopia. R. — V = $\frac{20}{8}$; L. — V = $\frac{10}{100}$. Hm. 1 25.

(178) RIGHT EYE—(Plate XII, Fig. 2, R.)

The posterior capsule presented a few fine striæ. Three start from the posterior pole, one going inward, one up, and one down. Five other shorter striæ are distributed about the periphery.

(179) LEFT EYE—(Plate XII, Fig. 2, L.)

The posterior capsule presented a close net-work of fine radiating striæ. They are grouped into ten bands or bundles, triangular in shape, with their apices pointing toward the pole, and their bases toward the equator. (Two smaller, shorter bundles, occur at the inner side.)

So sharply contoured were they, and so clear the lens, that a very good view of the fundus could be obtained through this lattice-work, and the clear strips between the bundles. This picture presents a remarkable similarity to the classical illustration of Koelliker, showing the post-crystalline vessels in injections of the developing eye. We have here almost a perfect survival of the fœtal vessels, as bloodless threads.

Group L—Persistent Canal.

The last group that we have to consider is one in which there remains, as a vestige of the hyaloid system, a delicate, nearly transparent, tubular sheath, passing through the center of the vitreous from the disc to the lens. This is regarded by some as the persistence of the delicate membranous lining of the canal of Cloquet, through which the hyaloid artery runs; and by others as the remains of the outer sheath of the vessel itself. This difference of opinion is due to our lack of absolutely decisive knowledge of this central canal, either in the embryo or the adult. According to Stilling, the sheath enveloping the hyaloid artery remains as an open tubular canal, after the vessel has disappeared. Manz and other authors hold this view, while Carreras and others hold that there is no really separate and distinct canal of Cloquet. The former view is most probably the correct one.

This group is not sharply limited. Some of the cases of flask-shaped cystic remains in Group C are analogous; and in several cases reported in other groups the persistent vessel is represented by a thin membranous expansion at the extremity joining the disc.

The anatomical examinations, as well as the ophthalmoscopic studies show that this canal consists of a delicate and nearly transparent membranous tube. This is much wider than the vessel ever is, being usually a millimeter, or a mm. and a half, or even more in diameter at its narrowest part—that is, about as wide as the disc itself. It usually terminates at either extremity by a funnel-shaped expansion even wider than this, so that at the posterior end the disc is usually well covered. This condition is, however, not always present; sometimes the sheath fades away toward the disc, and only a thin pointed extremity fixes it at this point; and even this may fade away so as not to be visible to the ophthalmoscope.

Anteriorly, this sheath may fade away in the same manner, and not reach the posterior surface of the lens. In rare instances this sheath may divide into two or even three branches, such division seeming to be sheaths that had been prolonged upon an equal number of branches, into which the hyaloid artery had divided, and which had formerly been inclosed by them. These are probably true sheaths of the vessel, for there seems to be no evidence that the canal of Cloquet proper subdivides in this manner. A good example of this is shown in the case of Holmes (190), illustrated in Plate XI, Fig. 1.

There is little doubt but that, in some instances at least, this canal remains patent during adult life. Stellwag mentions a case, at p. 134 of the American edition (4th) of his Treatise on Diseases of the Eye, "In which there was a thin, vessel-like, sharply demarcated column of blood, which ran from the optic papilla toward the center of the posterior capsule, and there expanded into a small disc-like extravasation. There were no walls to be found, however, in this blood column, and hence it was explained as an injection of Cloquet's canal, such as often really occurs in post-mortem injections made for anatomical purposes."

Galezowski notes a case where a very fair example of the persistence of the posterior portion of this canal had been observed in an infant; and three years later this had dwindled to a few shreds floating at the disc. From this he concludes that this condition is quite frequent in infancy, to usually disappear as the infant grows to childhood. This conclusion is hardly warranted from a single observation, especially when we consider how large have been the number of examinations of infants' eyes without this condition being noted.

It is interesting to note that in almost all of these cases the persistent canal is found in *both* eyes. In the ordinary forms of persistent artery, on the other hand, the remnant occurs in but *one* eye, in more than five-sixths of the cases. Why there should be this marked difference is not clear.

MANZ (*b*)—(Plate XII, Fig. 7).

(180) Young unmarried woman of 24 yrs.; died in the Freiberg Hospital. Her

eye had presented a dense central leucoma of the cornea, so that, ante-mortem, nothing could be seen of the fundus.

From the middle of the disc a short process (much resembling those frequently found in the ox's eye), projected into the vitreous. It was surrounded by a very delicate, transparent, tubular sheath, which passed forward through the center of the vitreous, to be inserted into the center of the posterior capsule. It was somewhat narrower in the center and slightly funnel-shaped at each extremity.

WECKER (b)—

(181-2) M. B——. Aet. 55. Came to consult about his glasses. Had hypermetropia of $\frac{1}{18}$, and $V = \frac{2}{3}$.

The ophthalmoscope revealed in each eye a dark strand running from the posterior pole of the lens to the optic disc. The point of attachment to the lens is perfectly circular; the strand is uniform, and of about the caliber of the primary branches of the central artery; it describes an S-shaped curve through the vitreous, and posteriorly is lost in the small, bright physiological cup, between the main stems of the central artery and vein. It undulates freely on movements of the eyeball. The vitreous is perfectly clear, and the fundus normal in each eye.

The strand is single contoured, and of a delicate transparency. With the oblique illumination the anterior extremity shows very faintly, it being so transparent. With the mirror alone, and the line of vision directed rather along the axis of the strand, it shows dark. With the indirect method and the disc in clear view, it gives the impression as if a glass rod traversed the vitreous between the observer and the pink disc; in fact, its attachment to the disc can only be made out by the closest observation and most careful focusing. With the direct method it shows a very delicate, but perfectly clear contour.

—— (c)—

(183-4) Woman of 45 yrs. Came on account of poor vision. Had dust-like opacities in each vitreous. A picture very similar to the above was seen in both eyes. The delicate tube was not inserted at the exact posterior pole, but somewhat downward and outward in each eye. The diameter was greater than that above, being slightly greater than the caliber of the main trunk of the central vein. The exact insertion into the disc could not be clearly made out, but W. was convinced that no blood-vessel projected into the posterior extremity at least.

The fundus was normal, so far as the clouded vitreous permitted this to be determined.

FLARER—

(185) Woman. Aet. 41. The ophthalmoscope revealed a grayish-white column passing from the posterior pole of the lens to the optic disc. It was immovable, with sharply outlined edges, but almost perfectly transparent. By examination in various ways it was seen to be a small canal, with very delicate and transparent walls. The posterior end was distinctly seen to be attached to the outer part of the disc; the anterior extremity could not be clearly traced to the lens, as the vitreous here was filled with numerous little floating opacities.

There was also a persistent pupillary membrane. $V = $ only $\frac{1}{20}$.

SCHINDELKA—

(186) Patient was a young girl. At the posterior pole of the lens there was noticed a white, triangular clump. From this there projected back a thin, translucent, sheath-like membrane—a sort of "neck" to the persistent remain. This narrow portion passed into a round cyst-like body, which much resembled a cysticercus. This then again narrowed. The disc was covered by the basal portion of a ribbed or ridged, cylindrical, tubular body, with a broadened base. This then narrowed somewhat in front into a thin strand, which passed bow-like through the vitreous to connect with the above structure on the lens.

GALEZOWSKI—

This author adds two cases of visible persistent canal.

(187) Case of young man. Aet. 17. Here the persistent canal sprang from the disc, and passed a short distance forward into the vitreous. It contained the atrophic vessel. This soon dwindled to a fine filament, which seemed to be attached to the posterior surface of the lens.

(188) Case of an infant. Aet. 18mos. Here the persistent canal was in the form of a membranous cone; with its base upon the papilla, and its apex found near, or fixed to the posterior pole of the lens. It is said to somewhat resemble Manz's case (Plate XII, Fig. 7).

It seems that the author saw this case three years later, and that this membranous sheath had dwindled to a few delicate shreds floating near the disc.

This he thinks occurs frequently.

(The above cases I was unable to quote from the original, and can not vouch for. The references I found seemed extremely imperfect, and somewhat hard to reconcile with one another.)

DESPAGNET—

(189) Patient came with asthenopia due to compound myopic astigmatism. There was present a persistent hyaloid canal—a delicate tubular sheath. No trace of the vessel could be detected in this tube. The sheath could not be traced back to the disc, so that the posterior attachment or mode of termination could not be clearly made out. This was due to the extreme delicacy of the sheath, and probably to the fact also that it really faded away at its posterior end near the disc.

HOLMES, C. R.—(Plate XI, Fig. 1).

I am indebted to Dr. C. R. Holmes, Oculist and Aurist to the Cincinnati Hospital, for the notes and sketch of the following case, observed in the practice of the late Dr. E. Williams, of Cincinnati.

(190) John W. W——. Aet. 48. Lost the right eye years before from a blow with a stick of wood. Came complaining of impaired V in the left eye, "a mist before the eye." The ophthalmoscope showed the disc and vessels normal, only the inferior temporal artery and vein being outlined with white bands.

At the macular region was a large oval, transverse area, over 1½ disc-diameters in height, and about 2½ disc-diameters in width. It was intensely pigmented, with some white atrophic patches, and a few vasular branches of small size. This was either a central coloboma, or a patch of choroiditis, probably congenital. I think most probably the latter, although the two conditions are essentially very analogous.

From the center of the disc, beginning with a narrow, conical point, there projected forward directly through the center of the vitreous, a hollow tubular strand having a diameter about ½ that of the disc. This was almost transparent, only veiling the vessels beneath, and of a bluish-gray tint, becoming darker as it passed further forward. Behind the lens it divided into three branches, all of which were darker than the trunk. The inner two seemed tubular, but the outer was much darker and looked solid. They all ended in fine dark points, which were not attached to the lens. The trunk, and especially the branches, floated freely about on movements of the eye.

The visual field was distinctly contracted, and there was a central scotoma corresponding to the macular patch. Slightly eccentric V was not impaired.

BAYER (b)—

(191) Married woman. Aet. 62. She had in the left eye $V = \frac{6}{12}$, with a corrected M. of $\frac{1}{10}$. The ophthalmoscope revealed an atrophic choroidal patch bounding the disc to the temporal side. From the middle of the disc there sprang a grayish, web-like, almost transparent tube. This passed forward through the middle of the vitreous with an S-shaped curve. It showed undulating movements on moving the eye. When near the posterior surface of the lens the tube divided at an acute angle, and the divisions seemed to be inserted into the posterior lens capsule. The artery was not detected within this tube. The author regards this division of the canal as a remarkable variation from the usual ending here with a funnel-like expansion, as described by Stilling, but the previous case shows that this is not unique.

OELLER—

(192) K. N——. Aet. 11. Had never noticed any defect, until on beginning target shooting, he found vision was defective in the right eye. Had slight H. and $V = \frac{5}{10}$. Left eye normal.

The ophthalmoscope showed in the R. eye a delicate, translucent tube, running through the center of the vitreous. It began upon the upper half of the disc, close to the division of the central artery, with a broad funnel-shaped base, whose horizontal diameter is greater than its vertical. This was of a dull greenish reflex, and appeared striated. Rapidly narrowing to the caliber of the central vein, it passed forward through the vitreous in an S-shaped curve. Near the lens, slightly to the inner side, it ended with a rounded extremity. From this there passed an extremely fine filament; but whether this was inserted into the posterior capsule could not be determined.

Looked at in line, the tube appeared as a flat, dark band; with the direct method it gave a delicate, dull greenish, gleaming contour. It made wide excursions on movements of the eye.

Vitreous and fundus were normal.

BOGDÁN—

(193) This author reports a case of persistent canal of Cloquet, visible with the ophthalmoscope. The details of the case I can not give, the Hungarian original not being accessible to me here.

The purely clinical features of this series of cases present nothing striking. Vision is in many of these cases not affected, and the anomaly is frequently only discovered on chance examination. In others, vision is affected to a greater or less degree, usually somewhat proportional to the extent of the persistent remains that are present. In many of the cases where a free strand floats in the vitreous, subjective sensations of shadows floating across the field of vision are complained of. This is usually not very troublesome, only Carreras-Arago (94), stating that in his case it caused vertigo.

Subsequent changes in these remains are seldom noted. Unterharnscheidt notes where such a strand had torn apart at its center, under the strain of a progressive myopia. Galezowski notes the case of a child, where a pretty well marked persistent canal had, after the lapse of three years, dwindled to some small floating shreds attached at the disc. In certain cases the sudden onset of floating shadows probably indicates the breaking loose of this strand from one of its attachments, and examination usually confirms this. This probably occurred in the case reported by Seely (154).

Secondary pathological changes seem to very seldom occur, and this is the more surprising when we consider how many of these cases have a floating strand rendering the vitreous fluid and continually agitated.

In the case of Vanlair (110), where the author thinks that this remain was the starting point of a vascular, malignant, intra-ocular tumor, the evidence is very inconclusive.

In the case reported by Nettleship (139), the numerous changes described, among which the degenerated vitreous and the thickened fibrous expansion spreading out from both ends of the hyaloid remain are the most important, were considered by him as taking origin in inflammatory changes starting from this persistent fœtal structure. We are disposed to place much reliance upon any views advanced by our able English colleague, and in this instance his conclusions have the additional weight of being based upon careful microscopical examination. However, this case forms really the only one in the series where this pathogenetic influence seems to be pretty well demonstrated. This rare result thus only more strikingly illustrates the customary absence of any subsequent degenerative or inflammatory changes, which may justly be claimed to have started from changes initiated by the presence of this abnormal structure. Thus the prognostic import of these remains is almost purely negative, and their presence not indicative of further future trouble.

Eversbusch is of the opinion that quite a large proportion of these cases, described as persistent hyaloid remains, are really pathological products. He thinks that in many instances an exudation into the vitreous, naturally following the line of least resistance, spreads along the open canal of Cloquet, and there organizing, produces these appearances which are so deceptively like persistent remains of the hyaloid artery.

This is one of those obscure questions that is difficult to prove either one way or the other.

My opinion, however, based upon a general study of the whole group, with regard to the general similarity amidst all the diversity, with regard to the visual acuity, and with regard to all the factors involved, does not coincide with his. But of course it is only a matter of individual opinion.

To my mind the strongest point in disproof of his view is the known fact that unquestioned vitreous exudations, either serous, plastic, hemorrhagic or purulent, show no tendency to take this path indicated. They occur indifferently in any part of the vitreous, just as likely to be peripheral as central.

Another point that bears in favor of their congenital nature, is their very frequent association with other anomalies of undoubted congenital character. The number of such anomalies in the foregoing group is really very striking, far in excess of any possible occurrence in any group of 174 individuals selected from any other sources, or at random.

Thus in Badal's case (127), there were dermoid tumors at the sclero-corneal junction.

There are three cases of hydrophthalmus, Haab (149) and Berthold (162 and 164). Two cases of microphthalmus, Hess (151) and Becker (141). There are two cases of cystic coloboma oculi, Wallman (117–18).

Of persistent pupillary membrane, there are the cases of Debierre (67), Sulzer (98), Vassaux (135), Becker (141) and Flarer (185). Of coloboma iridis, Wallman (117), Eversbusch (150) and Hess (151).

Of irideremia the cases of Pflueger (95 and 96–7), Oeller (163), Felser (167–8) and Ammon (173). A total of ten eyes.

Of congenital cataract, at least two cases, Larsen (129) and Ammon (152). Of lenticonus anterior, the case of Webster (175); of lenticonus posterior, the three cases of Ammon (152), Webster (155) and Meyer (158). Of coloboma lentis, the case of Gunn (122); and of ectopia lentis, the three cases of Gunn (122), Wecker (121) and Hess (151).

Of remnants of the mesoderm process at the floor of the vitreous, the cases of Bayer (63), Sulzer (98), Reuss (105), Wallman (117–18) and Eversbusch (150).

Of coloboma of the choroid there are several cases, Goldzieher (42), De Schweinitz and Randall (52—see Plate VIII, Fig. 1), Dimmer (55—see Plate VI, Fig. 1), Remak (111—see Plate V, Fig. 5; and 112—see Plate VIII, Fig. 2), Wallman (117) and Larsen (129). A central or macular coloboma existed in my case (86). Central congenital choroiditis in the two cases of Bayer (146—Plate XI, Fig. 2) and Holmes (190—Plate XI, Fig. 1).

Choroiditis occurred in many cases, most of which were probably congenital. Rocliffe (44), Randall (53), Guene (54), Dimmer (55 and 56), Reuss (61, 104 and 105), Hersing (65), Eversbusch (66), my cases (85 and 86), Perrin (93), Carter (99), Lang (102), Hirschberg (124), Brailey (140), Bayer (191), and some others (see the various plates).

Retinitis pigmentosa in Ulrich's three cases (15, 71 and 72). Anomalous, probably congenital, retinal pigmentation in the cases of Dimmer (55 and 56), Reuss (60 and 105). Retinal anomalies in the cases of Vassaux (135—see Plate I, Fig. 4) and Webster (175).

An "underlying conus" occurs in the cases of Remak (84—see Plate V, Fig. 6), my case (51—see Plate IX, Fig. 1), Sulzer (98) and Reuss (157). There are three cases of coloboma of the optic nerve, Goldzieher (42), Becker (141), and Reuss (60—see Plate VII, Fig 1). Bayer's case (146—Plate XI, Fig. 2) has also a congenital anomaly of the nerve.

In other words, the group presents a sum total of nearly 100 congenital anomalies, other than the persistent hyaloid arteries.

We can then sum up the cases as including 174 individuals, presenting a total of 199 examples of some variety of a persistence of some portion of the fœtal hyaloid system. · Thus in 25 of these cases the defect occurs in both eyes (6 of these I have not thought worth while to number separately in our tables).

What is rather striking is the fact that where this anomaly occurs in both eyes, it is usually so symmetrical that all these cases, with but two exceptions, have both eyes described under the same special group. These two exceptions are the cases of Little (16 and 134) and Reuss (61 and 157).

In 149 cases the anomaly occurs in but one eye.

The cases occurring in both eye are those of Schaumberg (9-10), Little (16-134), Randall (30-31, 32-33), Dimmer (55-56), Ulrich (71-72), DeBeck (17-50, 85-86, 176-177, 178-179), Reuss (61-157), Oettinger (74-75, 76-77), Ewers (88-89), Pflueger (96-97), Kipp (109), Wallman (117-118), Eversbusch (150), Webster (155), Oeller (163), Wilde (165, 166), Felser (167-168), Wecker (181-182, 183-184).

Of the 199 cases, 118 are examples of the persistent vessel or canal, 68 are examples of remnants at the disc—shreds, membranes, cysts or clumps, and 23 are examples of remnants at the posterior surface of the lens alone—capsular cataracts or striæ. (A few duplicated.)

———— ◆ ————

MEDICAL COLLEGE OF OHIO,
CINCINNATI, O., Sept., 1890.

BIBLIOGRAPHY.

AMMON (F. A. VON)—(a) "Klinische Darstellung der Krankheiten und Bildungsfehler des menschlichen Auges." (Theil III. Bildungsfehler.) Plate XV, Fig. 12.   Berlin.   1847...152

(b) The same.   Plate XIV, Fig. 5.   161

(c) The same.   Plate XIII, Fig. 4, 10, 11.   173

———— Graefe's Archiv für Ophthalmologie. pp. 151–55. Bd. IV, Abt I. 1858.

BADAL (Dr.)—"Gazette Hebd. des Sciences Medicales de Bordeaux." Tome 2. p. 728.   1880...127

BAYER (FR.)—(a) "Prager Medizinischer Wochenschrift." Bd. 6, No. 35. p. 342.   1881 ..145

(b) Prager Zeitschrift für Heilkunde. Bd. 4, p. 49.   1883.
....62, 63, 191

BECKER (OTTO)—(a) Sitzungsbericht der ophthalmologischen Gesellschaft. Heidelberg. (Zehender's Monatsbl. Augenheilkunde, Oct.—Dec., 1868.) p. 354.   1868.
....58, 59, 108

(b) Graefe und Sæmisch's "Handbuch der gesammten Augenheilkunde." Vol. 5, p. 285. Leipzig.   1875...141

BERGER (A. M.)—"Mittheilungen aus der augenärztlichen Praxis." p. 20. München.   1876.
....68, 87

BERGER (E)—(a) Zehender's Klinische Monatsblätter für Augenheilkunde. Vol. 20, p. 269.   1882.
....12, 13, 14

(b) Zehender's Klin. Monatsbl. für Augenheilkunde. Vol. 22, p. 284. 1884...174

BERTHOLD (E)—(a) Græfe's Archiv für Ophthalmologie. Bd. 17, Abt. I. p. 169.   1871...164

(b) Klinische Darstellung der Krankheiten des Auges. Vol. III, p. 67. 1882 ..162

BOCK—v. Wedl und Bock.

BOGDAN (A.)—Szemészet (Hungarian). p. 53.   1888...193

BRAILEY (WM. A.)—" Royal London Ophthalmic Hospital Reports " Vol. VIII. pp. 543–4.   1876.
.... 64, 140

CALLAN (PETER A.)—New York Medical Journal. Vol. 22, p. 43. July. 1875....90

CARRERAS-ARAGO (L.)—Hirschberg's " Centralblatt für praktische Augenheilkunde" Vol. 5, p. 44. (Report Milan Ophthalmological Congress, 1880. " Revista de Sciencias Medicales." No. 5, p. 205. 1881)   1881...94

CARTER (R. B.)—(a) Practical Treatise on Diseases of the Eye. Edited by Dr. John Green. p. 50. 8vo. Philadelphia.   1876....41

(b) Translations of the Ophthalmological Society of the United Kingdom. Vol. VI, p. 377.   1886....99

COWELL (GEO.)—Royal London Ophthalmic Hospital Reports. Vol. VI, p. 253 London.   1869 ...79

HOLMES (E. L.)—"Clinical Contributions." Archives of Ophthalmology. Vol. 10, p. 168. N. Y.   1881....43

KIPP (CHAS. J.)—(a) "Archives of Ophthalmology and Otology. Vol. III. p. 70. 1873. German edition, Vol. III, p. 190.   1874 ..109

(b)—Tenth Annual Report of the Newark, N. J. (U. S. A.) Eye and Ear Infirmary. p. 16 Newark.   1890...159

KOLLOCK (CHAS. W.)—The Medical News. Vol. 49, p. 456. Oct.   1886....39

KÖNIGSTEIN (L.)—Wiener Medizinische Wochenschrift. No. 44.   1884....46

LANG (W.)—Transactions of the Ophthalmological Society of the United Kingdom. Vol. 5, p. 141. London.   1885...102

LARSEN (M.)—Ungeschrift for Laeger (Danish). Vol. 20, p. 455. Copenhagen, 1875. Nagel's Jahresbericht über Ophthalmologie. Vol. 6, p. 185. 1875.
....128, 129

LAURENCE (J. Z.)—Ophthalmic Review (Old Series). Vol. II, p. 173. London.   1866...115

LIEBREICH (RICH.)—Zehender's Monatsblätter für Augenheilkunde. Vol. I, pp. 260 and 350.   1863...145
(Reported by Zehender)

LITTLE (W. S.)—Transactions of the American Ophthalmological Society. Vol. 3, p. 372. 18th meeting.   1882
....16, 80, 134

LORING (E. G.)—(a) Text-book of Ophthalmoscopy. Vol. I, p. 98.* Royal 8vo. New York.   1886....29

(b) The same. pp. 103-4.   ..113

McHARDY (M. M.)—(a) Transactions of the Ophthalmological Society of the United Kingdom. Vol. I, p. 217.   1881...125

(b) The same. Vol. IV, p. 352.   1884 ..126

MACKENZIE (W.)—A Practical Treatise on the Diseases of the Eye. p. 508. Third edition. 8vo. London. 1840. p. 564. Fourth edition. 8vo. Philadelphia.   1855...160

MAGNUS (H.)—Zehender's Klinische Monatsblatter für Augenheilkunde. Vol. 25, p. 204.   1887...107

MANZ (W.)—(a) "Das Auge der hirnlosen Missgeburten." Virchow's Archiv für pathologische Anatomie. Vol. 51, p. 313, pl. 2. figs. 1, 2 and 3. 1870..142

(b) "Missbildungen des menschlichen Auges." Graefe und Saemisch's Handbuch der gesammten Augenheilkunde. Bd. II, p. 98, fig. 6.   1875 ..180,

MEISSNER (PROF.)—"Zeitschrift für rationelle Heilkunde." III Reihe, I. p. 562.   1857....70

MEYER (F.)—Hirschberg's "Centralblatt für praktische Augenheilkunde" Bd. 12, p. 41.   1888...158

MOOREN (A.)—(a) Ophthalmiatrische Beobachtungen. p. 203. Berlin. 1867....91

(b) Fünf Lustren Ophthalmologischer Wirksamkeit. p. 292. Wiesbaden. 1882....92

MUELLER (D. E.)—" Mittheilungen aus der Praxis." Graefe's Archiv für Ophthalmologie. Bd. II, Abt. 2, p. 168.   1856 ..171

MUELLER (H.)—"Graefe's Archiv für Ophthalmologie." Bd. II, Abt. II, p. 65.   1856.

———" Polar-staar"—Verhandlungen der Würzburger med-phys. Gesellschaft. p. 159.   1858.

NETTLESHIP (E)—Reports of the Royal London Ophthalmic Hospital. Vol. VII p. 632.   1873 ..139

NOYES (H D.)—Report of the Fifth International Ophthalmological Congress, New York, 1876. p. 159. 8vo. N. Y.   1877...1-5

OELLER (J. N.)—Zur Aetiologie der cataracta polaris posterior congenita. Inaug. Dissertation. München. pp. 7 and 16. 1878.
....162, 192

OETTINGER (G. v.)—(a) "Dorpater Medizinische Zeitschift." Bd. II, p. 169. 1871.
....74, 75

(b) The same. Bd. II, p. 337. 1871.
....76, 77, 78

PERRIN (MAURICE)—Atlas des Maladies Profondes de l' Oeil. Pt. I, Ophthalmoscopie. Plate 25, fig. 1. Imp. 8vo. Paris. 1879....39

PFLUEGER—Bericht der Universitäts Augenklinik in Bern für das Jahr 1882. p. 38. Bern. 1884.
....95, 96, 97

PICQUE (LUCIEN)—Anomalies de Développement et Maladies Congénitales du Globe de l' Oeil. Thèse d' Agrégation. 4to. pp. 288 to 307. Paris. 1886.

RANDALL (B. ALEX.)—Transactions of the American Ophthalmological Society. Vol. 4, p. 116. 24th meeting. 1888.
....30, 31, 32, 33, 34, 36, 37, 52, 53

REMAK (Dr.)—Hirschberg's Centralblatt für praktische Augenheilkunde. Vol. 9, p. 9. 1886.
....84, 111, 112

REUSS (A. v.)—"Ophthalmologische Mittheilungen aus der Zweiten Universitäts-Augenklinik in Wien. II. Abt. p. 5. 1886.
....60, 61, 101, 103, 104, 105, 130, 157

ROCLIFFE (W. C.)—Transactions of the Ophthalmological Society of the United Kingdom. Vol. 7, p. 226. 1887....44

RUMSZIEWICZ—Medycyna. No. 27. (Polish.) 1882.
....132, 133

SAEMISCH (THEO.)—(a) Zehender's Klinische Monatsblatter für Augenheilkunde. Vol. 1, p. 258. 1863...119

(b) The same. Vol. 7, p. 304. 1869.
....69, 153

SATTLER (H.)—Becker's "Pathologie und Therapie des Linsensystems."—Graefe u. Saemisch's Handbuch d. gesammten Augenheilkunde. Vol. 5, p. 237. Leipzig. 1875...136

SCHAUMBERG (C. F.)—Casuistischer Beitrag zu den Missbildungen des Auges. Inaug. Diss. P. 24, pl. 3. Marburg. 1882.
....9, 10, 11, 23, 24

SCHINDELKA (Dr.)—Wiener Medizinischer Blatt. VII, No. 12, p. 357. 1884...186

SCHMIDT-RIMPLER (H.)—Graefe's Archiv für Ophthalmologie. Bd. 23, Abt. 4. p. 180, pl. VI, figs. 2 and 3. 1877.
....7, 8

SEELY (W. W.)—Transactions of the American Ophthalmological Society. Vol. 3, p. 344. Eighteenth meeting. 1882..154

SNELL (S.)—Transactions of the Ophthalmological Society of the United Kingdom Vol. 4, p. 349 1884 ..131

STELLWAG (C. VON CARION)—Treatise on the Diseases of the Eye. Translated by Roosa, Bull and Hackley. p. 134, fig. 26. 8vo. N. Y. 1873...106

STILLING (J.)—Graefe's Archiv für Ophthalmologie. Bd. 14, Abt 3, p. 260. 1868.

STÖR (Dr.)—Zehender's Klinische Monatsblätter für Augenheilkunde. Vol. III, p. 24. 1865...123

STREATFIELD (J. F.)—London Lancet. I. p. 308. February. 1882...100

SULZER (Dr.)—Zehender's Klinische Monatblätter für Augenheilkunde. Vol. 26, p. 425. 1888....98

TANGEMAN (C. W.)—Archives of Ophthalmology. Vol. 17, p. 270. 1888....147

TOUSSAINT v. Zehender (b.)

ULRICH (RICH.)—Zehender's Klinische Monatsblätter für Augenheilkunde.
Vol. 20, p. 240.   1882.
....15, 71, 72

UNTERHARNSCHEIDT—Zehender's Klinische Monatsblätter für Augenheilkunde.
Vol. XX, p. 449.   1882 ..116

VANLAIR (C.)—Archives de physiologie normale et pathologique. Tome VII,
p. 459.   1880 ..110

VASSAUX (G.)—"Archives d' Ophthalmologie." Vol. III, p. 502, pl. VI. 1883...135

WALLMANN (H.)—Zeitschrift der Gesellschaft der Aerzte zu Wien. p. 446.
No. 28   1858.
....117, 118

WEBSTER (D.)—"Clinical Contributions." Archives of Ophthalmology and
Otology. Vol. 4, p. 384. N. Y.   1874.
....155, 175

WECKER (L. de)—(a) Annales d' Oculistique." T. 53, p. 65.   1865...121

(b) Zehender's Klinische Monatsblätter fuer Augenh'de. Vol. 7, p. 210. 1869.
....181, 182

(c) "Graefe's und Saemisch's Handbuch der Gesammten Augenheilkunde.
Bd. IV, p. 702.   1876.
....183, 184

WEDL (C.) AND BOCK (E.)—Pathologische Anatomie des Auges. Mit Atlas.
Fig. 193. Wien.   1886 ..134

WILDE (W. R.)—An Essay on the Malformations and Congenital Diseases of
the Organs of Sight. pp. 129 and 131. 8vo. London.   1862.
....165, 166, 172

ZEHENDER (W.)—(a) "Klinische Monatsblätter fuer Augenheilkunde." Vol. I,
p. 259.   1863...144

(b) (Case of Dr. Toussaint.) Klinische Monatsblätter fuer Augenheilkunde.
Vol. I, p. 349.   1863 ..120

' ADDENDA.

Since the foregoing was in type there has come to hand an inaugural dissertation upon this subject; containing a careful report of a case with the defect occurring in both eyes. It belongs under the ordinary forms as collected in Groups E and G.

FUCHS (ROBERT). Ein Fall von doppelseitiger Arteria hyaloidea persistens. Inaugural Dissertation. Strassburg. 1890.

A case is also noted that had escaped observation up to this time:

SCHLEICH (G.) "Die Augen der Idioten der Heil-und Pflege-Anstalt Schloss Stetten in Württemberg." Zehender's Klin. Monatsbl. für Augenheilkunde. p. 452, XXIII. 1885.

Man, Aet. 21. From the disc-center of the left eye projected a whitish, conical process. From the point of this there sprang some fine vessels, or fibres, which passed forwards into the vitreous, without reaching its anterior portion. V. was much reduced. There was H. of 2 D. The right eye normal.

The case is inadequately described; but seems to really belong to Group E.

INDEX OF THE PLATES.

Plate I.

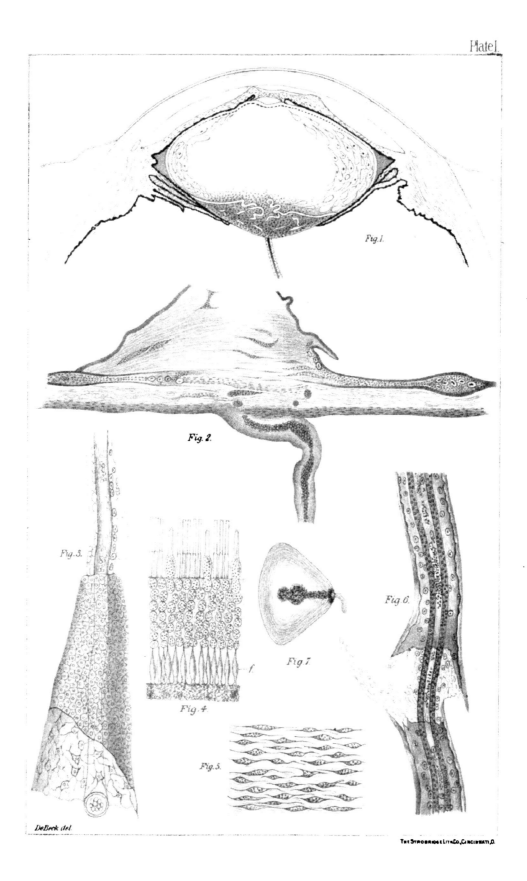

Fig. 1.

Fig. 2.

Fig. 3.

Fig. 4.

Fig. 5.

Fig. 6.

Fig 7.

f.

DeBeck del.

THE STROBRIDGE LITH.CO., CINCINNATI, O.

Plate II.

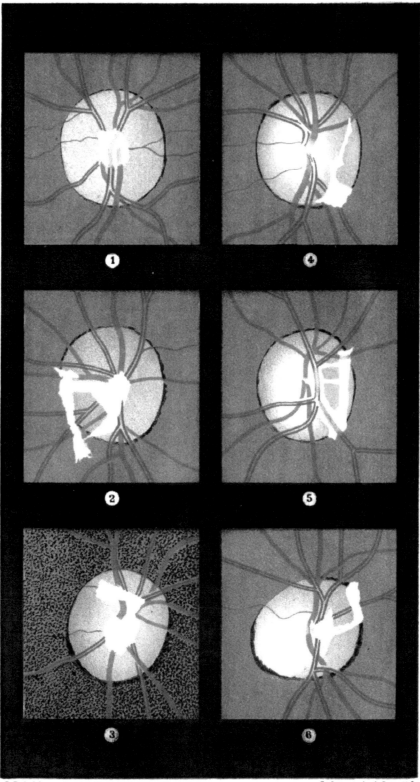

Plate III.

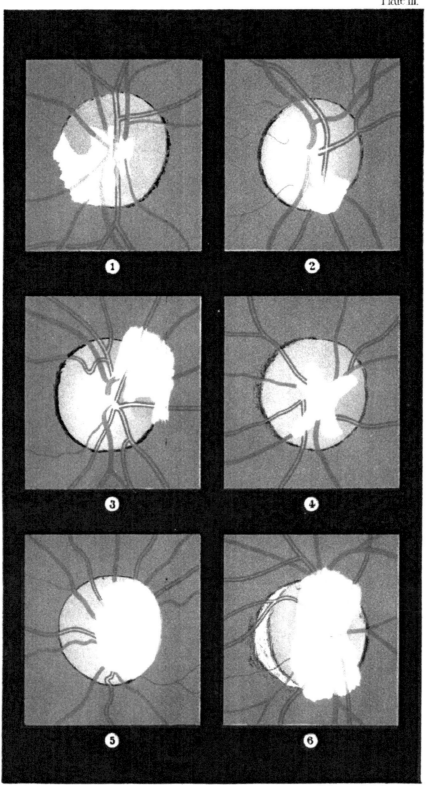

Plate IV.

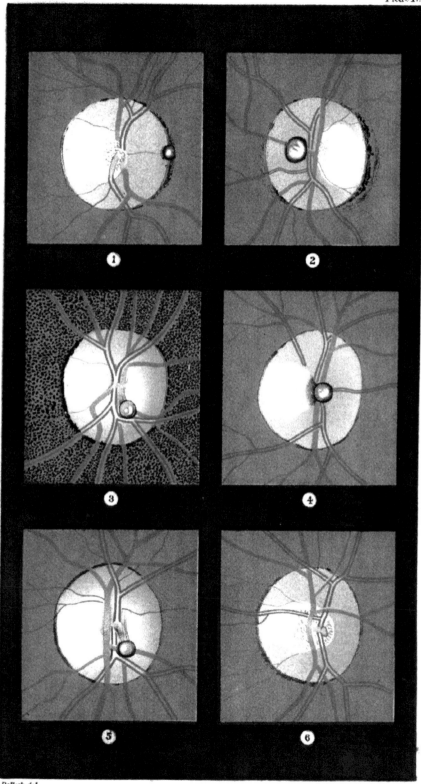

Plate V.

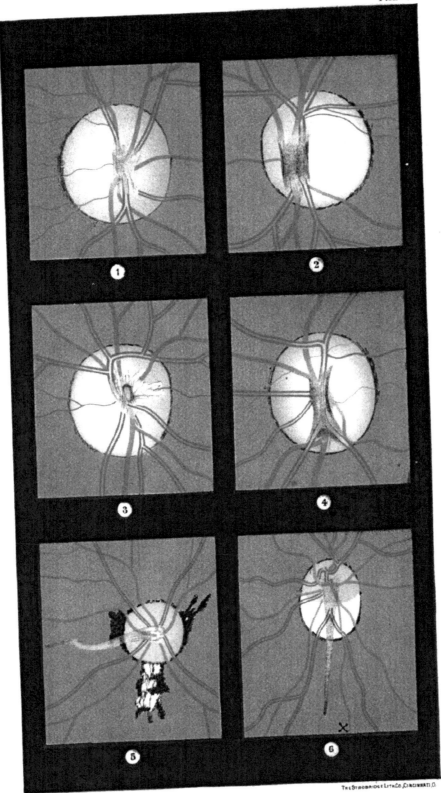

DeBeck del.

The Strobridge Litho.Co.,Cincinnati,O.

Plate VI.

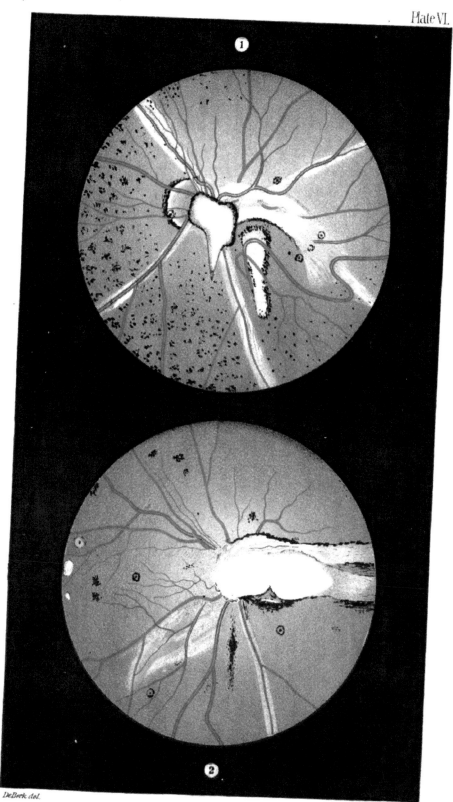

Plate VII.

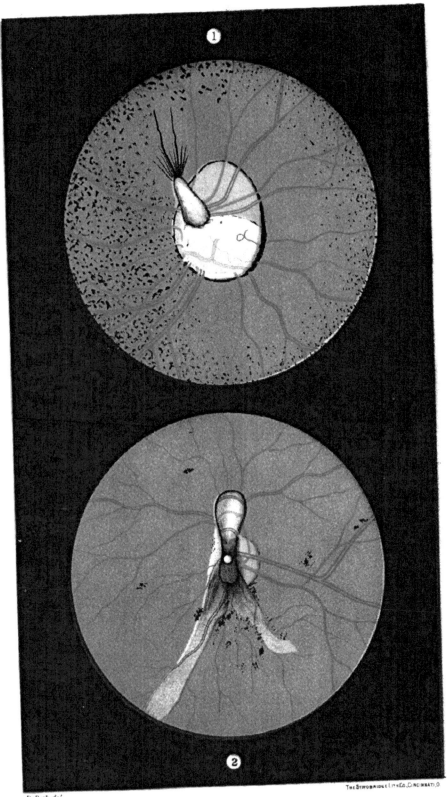

Plate VIII.

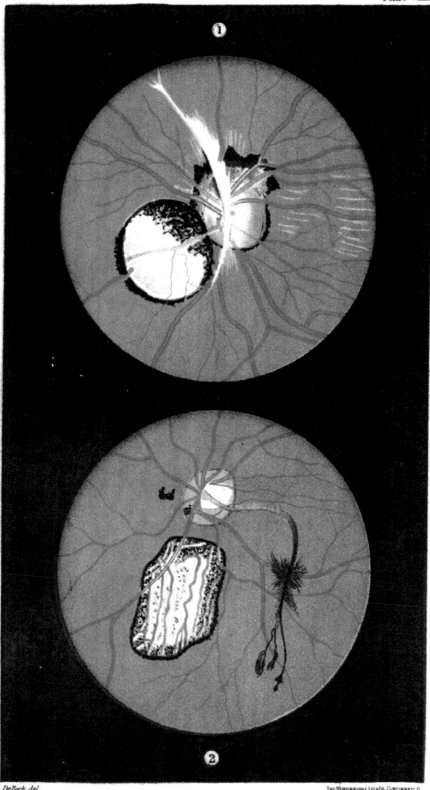

DeBeck del.

THE STROBRIDGE LITH.CO., CINCINNATI, O.

Plate IX.

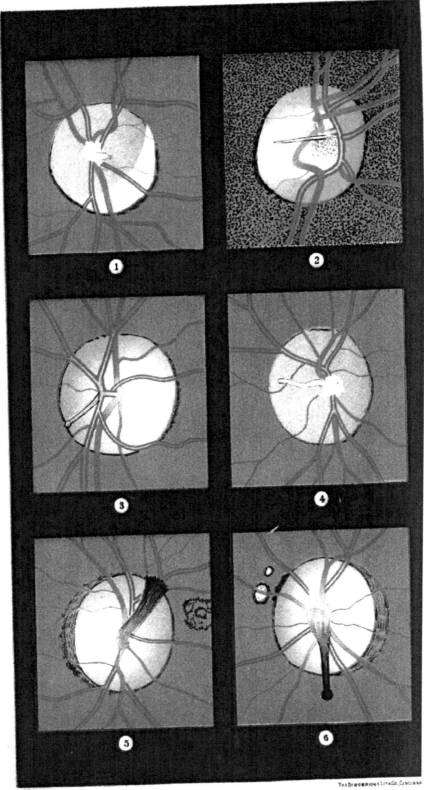

Plate X.

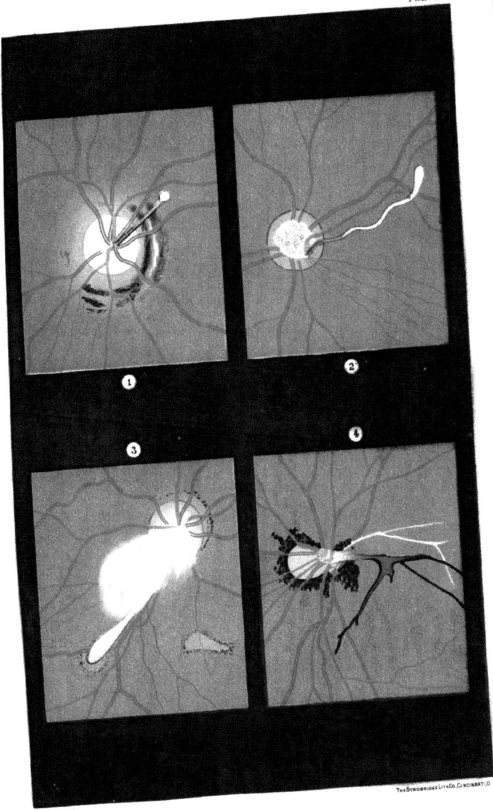

DeBeck del.

TheStrobridgeLith.Co.Cincinnati,O

Plate XI.

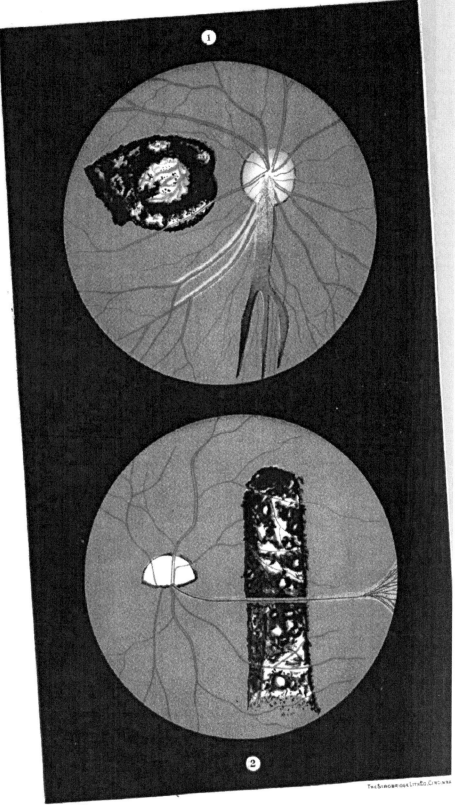

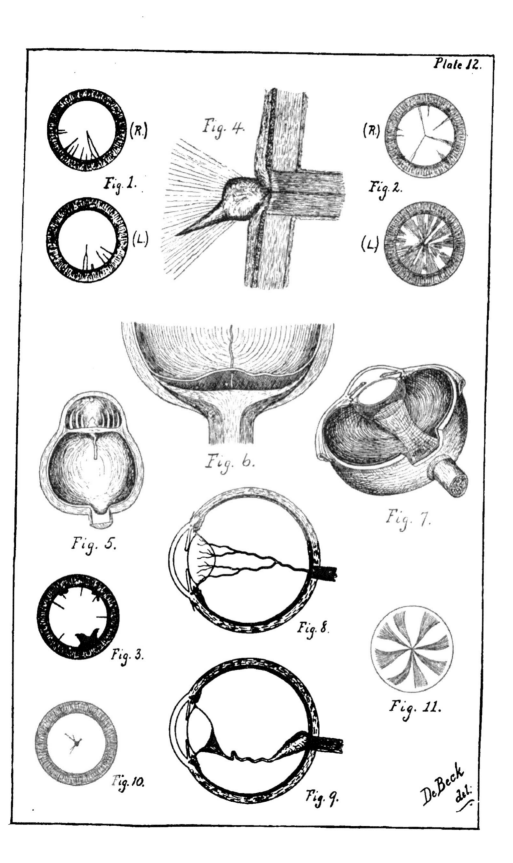

Plate 12.

(R.)

Fig. 1.

(L.)

Fig. 4.

(R.)

Fig. 2.

(L.)

Fig. 6.

Fig. 5.

Fig. 7.

Fig. 3.

Fig. 8.

Fig. 11.

Fig. 10.

Fig. 9.

De Beck del.

CPSIA information can be obtained at www.ICGtesting.com
Printed in the USA
LVOW030213300412

279553LV00003B/27/P

9 781179 047829